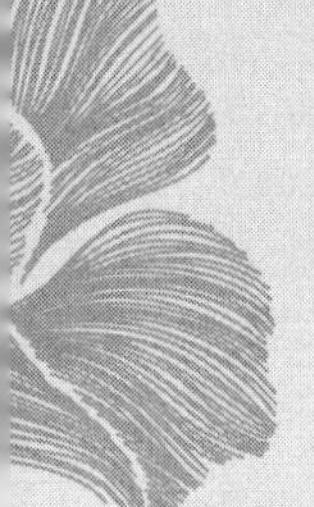

collide

Running into healing when life hands you hurt

willow weston

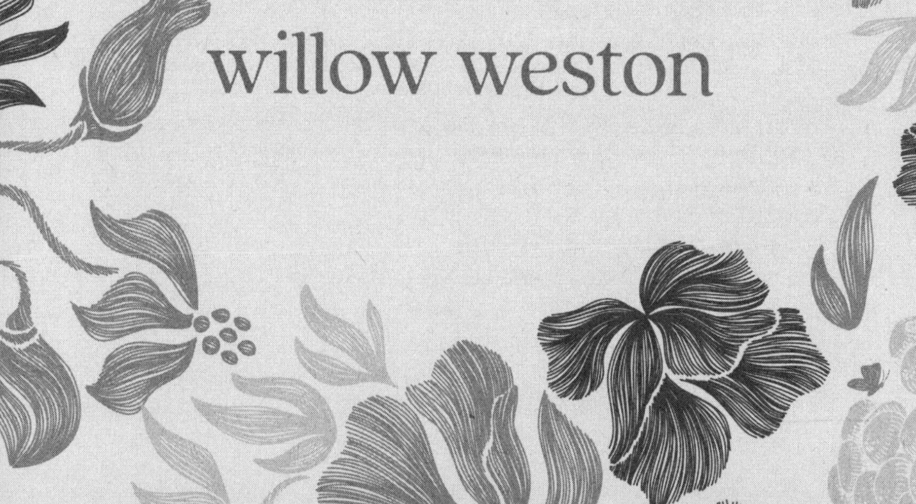

Visit Tyndale online at tyndale.com.

Visit Tyndale Momentum online at tyndalemomentum.com.

Visit the author online at willowweston.com.

Collide: Running Into Healing When Life Hands You Hurt

Cover design by Eva M. Winters

Interior design by Brandi Davis

Published in association with the literary agency of Embolden Media Group, PO Box 953607, Lake Mary, FL 32795-3607.

Library of Congress Cataloging-in-Publication Data

A catalog record for this book is available from the Library of Congress.

ISBN 979-8-4005-1138-7

Printed in the United States of America

32 31 30 29 28 27 26
7 6 5 4 3 2 1

Collide is a soul-stirring invitation to healing. Willow writes with vulnerability and insight, offering women a lifeline of hope as they walk through life's heartbreaks. This book will meet you in your pain and gently lead you to the Healer.

BOB GOFF
New York Times bestselling author, speaker, and coach

In *Collide*, Willow Weston, through her own vulnerable storytelling and honest teaching, has offered us not only a path to healing but a process to deepen our faith in a loving and kind God, a journey to take that will grow us and change us, and an opportunity to run the race marked out for each of us. What a gift of a book.

ANNIE F. DOWNS
New York Times bestselling author of *That Sounds Fun*

In a world where it's easy to hide the hard, Willow is choosing to be raw and vulnerable out loud, and it's transforming an entire generation of women. I'm just grateful to be able to see it up close through the Collide conference year after year! I can't wait to see the fruit of her bravery on paper.

TONI COLLIER
Author, preacher, and podcast host

Willow has an infectious love for God, His Word, and other people that permeates her life. If you have the privilege of being around her—whether through her teaching, her writing, or simply waiting beside her in line at a coffee shop—you'll encounter genuine joy!

LISA HARPER
Author, Bible teacher, and host of *Back Porch Theology*

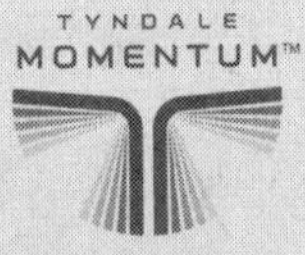

A Tyndale nonfiction imprint

To the one whose life has handed you hurt—
may these pages hand you healing.

contents

Introduction *ix*

Part 1: Running Away from Pain

1. Hiding in Closets *3*
2. Taught *9*
3. We Don't Move On *17*
4. Not Dealing Is Not Healing *29*
5. A Wounded Collision *35*
6. Left More Whole Than Broken *47*

Part 2: Running Into a Healing God

7. I'm Not Fines *55*
8. Drunkards, Gluttons, and Swingers *65*
9. Wanting to Be Wanted *75*
10. Absence Makes the Heart *85*
11. Rescue *97*
12. Thirst Traps *107*
13. If You Hads *119*
14. Reckless *129*
15. The Over and Over Again *139*
16. Getting Unstuck *149*
17. The Power of B *159*
18. Get Out of the Boat *171*
19. The Ultimate Wounded Collision *181*

Part 3: Running Toward Pain to Bring Healing

20. Get Off the Bus *191*

21. The Park Bench *197*

22. Make It Count *203*

23. Always *209*

24. The Yellow Butterflies *217*

25. Mended and Restored *225*

A Blessing *237*

Amazed and Amen *241*

Discussion Questions *243*

Notes *247*

Acknowledgments *253*

About the Author *257*

introduction

Dear friend,

You and I have been through a lot. We have experienced some joyous joys but also some tremendous loss and pain. We have run into hurting people who hurt us. And I'm afraid we haven't always been invited to heal in ways that truly heal. If we don't get healing for what hurt us, our wounds start to wound and wound and wound.

Our wounds begin to speak. Our experiences, conversations, and memories have a voice, and they start to tell us who we are, who others are, and who God is. Our view of ourselves, others, and God can become so very wounded.

We walk into job interviews, parties, churches, teams, first dates, and committees expecting to be hurt again, which wreaks havoc on our lives. We self-protect by controlling, hiding, shutting down, and putting up walls. Some of us build such high walls that they put the Great Wall of China to shame. Nobody will ever climb them. And if someone *tries* to climb our walls, we will Taser them with our pain. That oughta keep them out!

Wounds that haven't experienced repair can lead to self-sabotage. This is the sad story of my life, and maybe yours too. We quit before we get fired. We dump before we get dumped. We withdraw before we get rejected. We break up with the cool kids club before they can break up with us. We live small so we aren't disappointed by dreaming big.

In all this pain, we look for easy versions of pleasure or safety or busyness with our deep-seated hurt. We turn to Cheetos and red wine and boobs and boob tube—anything we can to avoid our pain.

Our wounds can find us trying so hard to convince others that we are worthy. We sign up for every board, every volunteer opportunity, every cause. We close more deals and drive flashier cars. We host parties that we hope are supercool so people think we are too. Sometimes we pretend we are nice when we don't feel nice. We laugh at jokes we don't think are funny. We say yes when we want to say no. We don't stand up for what *is* right because we want to be *in* the right with those we know are wrong.

Before long, the hurt from our past begins to mess with our present. We stop trusting people, assuming they will hurt us, reject us, or betray us. We stop taking risks in community, and we begin growing roots of bitterness. We become full of unforgiveness, and we drink its poison.

We let our pain tell us false stories about other people's motivations, and we act on our assumptions. This leads to ghosting, friendship breakups, conflict, divorce, and empty seats at family get-togethers. We start blaming others, and we start blaming God for our pain and for not taking it away. Before we realize it, we've become the father we despised, the boss we'd hate working for, the friend we're annoyed by. Our marriages experience mutual destruction, our friendships are damaged by deep-seated insecurity, and our kids are handed wounded patterns with their breakfast. We pass the baton of hurt on to our children, who pass it on to their children and their children's children. We see history repeat itself, and what we see, we don't like.

Pain can be ravaging our lives, and still we fail to pause for repair, reach out for help, or travel back to the origin of our wounds. We try to move on like that thing that happened didn't sting, *but it stings*. Like that cut only needs a Band-Aid, *but it still bleeds*. Like that run-in didn't tear us apart, *but it did*. You can say, "It's nothing," for fifty years. You can make it small, but it sure is pestilent. You can ice it over with gin and tonics. You can stuff it away for safekeeping and try to forget it's in there. But the thing is, wounds that aren't healed continue to wound and wound and wound.

I don't have to be a psychologist or have lots of letters after my name to understand pain. I've learned from the school of life. I grew up in a hippie commune, a school bus, a houseboat, and a famous café with quirky, hurting, religionless folk. I was raised by a wild and crazy alcoholic mother who left me alone all too often while she chased her longings. Every once in a while she'd bring those longings home, and what I experienced wrecked me. My dad was nowhere to be found for years, and his absence left a hole in my heart that found me chasing my own longings. The pain that was handed to them was passed on to me. Absence and neglect, abuse and addiction, secrets and silence, instability and feeling all alone in the world taught me grit, resilience, and survival techniques, sure. But let's be real, mostly it taught me what pain feels like.

I bet you know pain too.

I have learned that if our wounds go unhealed, they will collide with others' woundedness and cause more wounds. We are in desperate need of a new kind of collision.

And I have found that healing collision possible in Jesus. So I want to tell you about this Jesus I have been colliding with, the One who is healing me, who wants to heal you too.

Jesus doesn't run away from pain—He runs toward it. When you look at Him in the New Testament, you see that every time He collides with someone, they are left more whole than broken. In my own agonizing pain, I invited a few friends, who then invited a few more friends, and I have since witnessed firsthand thousands of women colliding with Jesus and experiencing the healing they've longed for. I have been inviting people to collide with Jesus now for more than twenty-five years, and I have seen the power of what happens in a person's life when they receive permission to be real about their pain and then take it to Jesus. He is, after all, the One who can handle it and heal it. So let me grab your hand, and let's go to the One who can do something about all this pain. The more you and I collide with Jesus, the more whole we become.

This story is for you if you have been wounded and long for healing. If you were expected to move on but you never did . . . if you had to be the parent but you were the kid . . . if you got hurt loving someone who was supposed to love you. If you're triggered by a knock on the door, by the mention of a name, by the mean girls who happen to be adults, I see you.

This story is for you if you think God wants nothing to do with you because you are too messy for Him. If you feel broken and want to be put back together again . . . if you hoped you'd be in a better place by now but you just aren't . . . if you *still* feel angry, bitter, and disappointed . . . if you cry at Christmas and you don't know why . . . if you wonder where God has been in all your pain . . . this book is for you. And as frightened as I was to write these pages, they are for me too.

I invite you to run into the One who brings wholeness to all this woundedness. The One who changed me and changes me, and who can change you too. When He collides with us, we are never the same, and neither are the people we run into.

So if your past is still haunting your present . . . if you have been in self-protective mode for way too long and it's hurting you more than protecting you . . . if you wanted your story to write differently than it has . . . I did too. Let's write a new one.

Willow Weston

part 1

running away from pain

1

hiding in closets

One ordinary Wednesday, I got a knock on the door that sent me into total panic. I looked through the peephole, and as though I were in grave danger, I grabbed my baby girl, sprinted up the stairs, and hid in a closet.

Now, I need to hand you just a wee bit of context so you don't assume that I panic *every* time someone shows up at my house. Countless teens have practically grown up in our home. Kids walk in without knocking and open our fridge without asking. We have hosted a million events with Mentos-and-Coke tricks, toilet paper shenanigans, Nerf gun wars, and chubby bunny competitions.

Our house is *that* house.

We've had cooking classes instructed by my amazing food blogging friend Sarah, theology nights taught by our genius friend Johnny, and milkshake and movie nights instigated by our old roomie Ron. We've hosted bridal showers, puppy parades, kidney donor celebrations, and

The Office Olympic parties. (There was also the classy versus trashy party that got me in big trouble, but we can talk about that another time.)

People show up at our door in need all the time. There was the jilted bride, the man who cheated on his wife, the orphaned college kid, and the suicidal grocery checker. We've opened our rooms to college interns, traveling missionaries, people trying to put their marriages back together, and lost souls with no family to take them in.

It's a revolving door, so a knock doesn't usually phase me.

You should also know that I am a functioning woman. Like, I shower. I make decisions. I lead people. I can control the remote, but I can also let someone else control it. I do everyday things without getting spooked by spiders, clowns, or dirt. I have friends I've had for decades, and I don't try to one-up them with how much sex I have, how big my diamond is, how front-row my T-Swift concert tickets are, or how small my appetite is. Mainly because I don't have most of those things, but still. Like, I'm not the chick-looking-all-calm-but-I've-come-up-with-four-ways-to-kill-you-in-my-head. I do yell a lot in pickleball. It's the best part of my game. I can be very feisty, that's true.

But I'm not a crazy mom. Well, not exactly. I mean, I did ask my husband to return to the hospital about two minutes after leaving with our newborn. I yelled, "Go back!! We have noooo idea what we're doing!" And I meant GO BACK.

This running into a closet dealio happened when Hurt knocked on my door. I had just quit my full-time ministry job and was trying to rock the stay-at-home-mom life. Everyday life looked like potty training and blowouts, breastfeeding and nipple cream, Target runs and nap time. It also looked like me going to bed every night wondering if I had done enough, taught enough, been enough. Maybe you do that too?

Yeah, I mean, I fretted that I might mess up my kids. (And you might be thinking, *Yeah, chick, you will. You're hiding in a closet with your baby.*) But from the moment I got pregnant, I longed to give my kids what I didn't get.

Maybe that's why I signed up for every mommy-and-me class, volunteered in my kids' classrooms, made homemade baby food, and read a million parenting books. Maybe that's why we went to the zoo, the children's museum, the aquarium, and church. Maybe my longing to give my kids what I didn't have is why every single night I sang songs and prayed prayers and said good night to everything and the moon. Maybe it's why I lay in bed with them when they were scared, held them when they cried, and invited them to feel all their feels. Their pain, their anger, their worry—all of it mattered.

That day at the front door, all my old emotions came flooding back. You'd think a serial killer was on my porch, or a religious guy selling me his heaven, or an ex-boyfriend begging me back. But nope. There, on the other side of the door, wearing denial like the tattered Hawaiian shirt on her back, stood my *mother*, showing up to be super grandma.

The moment I saw her, I ran like heck.

I ran like we all run. We get as far away from pain as we need to so we don't have to face it *or* feel it. We attempt to escape our own baggage, our own anxiety and emotions, and, well, our own issues because maybe, just maybe, they will all go away. Maybe if we get away from our reality, it won't be real. Maybe if we run for the hills, that person can't hurt us again. Maybe if we stuff down how we really feel, the peace we long for will finally show up. Maybe if we hide, our struggles will stop knocking.

Bella and I hid on the floor of that cramped closet together.

When you're hiding in a closet shushing your baby, there are a few things going on.

One: You're waiting for something bad to happen, and you are embarrassed your baby is seeing that you are a fraidy-cat, because nothing bad *is* actually happening.

I mean, for the love of all things holy, pull yourself together, Willow. (My self-talk has always been soooo helpful.) *This isn't what mature thirty-year-old Christian moms do.*

Two: You are horrified that you may be a wreck of a mom and may have lost all sense of logic. You remember that your infant is not psychoanalyzing you because she doesn't have that capacity . . . yet.

(Noooo, that comes in college, when you'll have to pay for tuition *and* therapy.)

And three: You just hope your little one won't start crying and alert your mother that you are actually inside, hiding from her.

My mom wasn't going to walk in and "hurt" me, I kept reminding myself. *What kind of mom will I be, and how will this hurt my daughter if this becomes our story?*

By now, Mom had been knocking for a while. I held my baby girl in my arms, hoping to wait her out. The knocking finally stopped, and breaking through the panic and paralysis, I heard something else: *This is an invitation into further healing.*

I knew this voice. It was God. I didn't have to come out for Him to find me. He met me right there in the closet. He was right. I needed more healing. With just one knock on the door, I could be triggered right back into being that little girl, full of fear, hiding to protect herself. God had already done so much healing in me since I handed Him my life, but here I was, needing Jesus to run into my mess, again.

Again?

Again.

Every closet is an invitation. Every trigger, every broken heart, every lie uncovered, every altercation, every walk-in absent of peace is God's request for our presence. It is there that God invites. His love can't bear to watch us shaking in the pain of old wounds, hushing our baby, inflicting new wounds. His love won't leave us there. It's often in these stuck places that we experience a real and personal, living and compassionate God, showing up and helping us get unstuck.

So I looked down at my sweet, precious Bella and chose to be brave for the both of us. Still uncertain and shaky, I held my baby girl in one arm, took a deep breath, and stretched for the door with the other. With all the guts I could muster, I walked out of that closet in search of help.

2

taught

You and I deal with pain the way we were taught to. Whether we knew it or not, our family of origin schooled us on how to handle our hurt. We became disciples of "Pick yourself up by the bootstraps," of "Chin up, buttercup," of "Pray it away," of "Ignore it and it will go bye-bye."

It wasn't like our parent people sat us down with a whiteboard and mapped out a plan for how we should deal with pain, but they certainly showed us by how they dealt with their own pain, and ours. Their avoidance mentored our avoidance. Their hyperfixation and fearmongering told us exactly how to handle hard things. The spiritual platitudes they tried for whisking pain away invited us to try them too. Their need to get us to feel anything but pain told us that we should escape pain at all costs by turning to cheap fixes to numb it all. Their inability to be real guided us to be more comfortable with acting like we are OK than with actually doing the work to become OK.

When I was in fifth grade, my mom and I were held hostage on a second-story deck in the middle of the night by a man on a rampage. I stood outside next to my bruised and bloody mother, who was stripped bare in the freezing cold, while John stood inside watching us suffer.

That night, they had been fighting. He dragged her—naked—up and down the staircase, and rug burns branded her skin stair by stair. She yelled desperately, but nothing she said and nothing I said had any power to stop his rage.

His hands—the hands that had taught me how to carve my first pumpkin, how to play "Every Good Boy Does Fine" on the clarinet, how to put a napkin on my lap, and how to make the chef's special—were now instruments of torture. John, the only present father figure I had known, had become a monster.

I paced.

I still pace.

They'd been drinking, which was not out of the ordinary. When they drank, it was always too much, and even then I knew that. Other times, they were strong, kind, fun, good-parent people. But not this night. No, this night he was angry, and she was a drunken mess.

I was in the way.

I still feel in the way.

I couldn't bear watching her be dragged around like a rag doll. So I mustered up as much nine-year-old courage as I could find and tried to match his mean mug with mine. Foolishly brave, I got up in his face to protect my mother, or at least give her a break.

"Leeeeave.

Myyyy.

Mooomm.

Aloooonne!"

John responded to me with the same anger he had for her. He

made sure I felt his fury and my powerlessness. He turned his rage to the furniture, burning and breaking things. Like an arsonist in his own home, like fuel doused on deadly flames, his fury became a wildfire that would consume us all.

As if this wasn't enough, he locked us outside on the second-story deck, holding us captive to his anger. We would have to beg the man who had just beaten us to let us back in, and when he did, he would be the hero. Either that or we would have to find another way to escape this terror. I looked over at my mother.

Shivering cold in fear, I wanted to scream for someone to save us. Anyone, any neighbor, any passerby, *anyone*. My buddies lived right next door. But my mom was muted in horror. The quiet did feel calming, like maybe there was a chance this torment was over. But on the inside, I was still screaming. *How can they hear us if we stay quiet?*

I looked at my bruised and naked mother, hoping for a cue. *Couldn't we just scream?*

Mom did not look at me.

She stayed silent.

So I stayed silent.

She was my teacher. I was her student.

I wanted safety, but I learned it's safer not to let anyone know you need it.

At some point that night, the valiant, violent John opened the door and let me and my naked mother back in from the freezing cold. I walked through the living room, past the woodstove that now housed the ashes of our things, up the stairs that bruised my mom, and into my bedroom. My little hippie princess bed was wrecked. My shelves were knocked down, my toys scattered across the room. My ladybug record player, broken. All the shattered pieces hinted at an old life that now felt like play and pretend.

When morning came, we frantically moved what was left of our belongings out of John's house to flee for safety. It was Valentine's Day, and I can still see the cards I had excitedly made for my classmates strewn across the dirty February snow. A handful of cards made it into our old blue truck. Some were crumpled. Others looked ready to deliver a "Be mine" message as if they had no other story to tell. I looked down and saw Heather's and Clayton's valentines, right along with the rest of them. In the hurry to pack our stuff, I remember thinking, *How can I only bring cards to* some *friends and not others?*

I was so looking forward to going to the school party. I wanted to escape into the normalcy of Valentine's Day—the no-work kind of school day, the lollipops and sugar cookies, the special note from the special boy. But those cards had seen something awful and ugly.

They shouldn't tell their secrets to other children.

The conversations that day between my mother and me did not revolve around how we were feeling. No one asked, "How are you doing? Are you scared? Do you need to talk?" There was never an invitation to process the pain. There *was* an invitation to push past it.

I don't remember engaging with the reality of our story, but I remember problem-solving how we would tell it.

"What happened to your eye?" they would ask.

"I got in a bike accident," I would say.

I was taught to be silent, to not talk about what was really going on, and if ever asked, I was coached to tell a different story than the one that had actually happened. I wonder . . . What were you taught? Did you learn to dismiss your own pain or someone else's? Were you taught that your feelings don't matter? Were you told it was *all* your fault, so that now you believe you deserve pain? Or maybe you were made to believe that God can't handle your wounds because someone who represented Him couldn't? Were you trained that crying is weak and so is asking for help? Did you learn to be "tough"?

I once was leading a room full of women leaders at a retreat, and I invited them to take turns sharing a time they had felt wounded and needed God's healing. One of the smartest, kindest, most beautiful young women you could ever meet piped up. She had an amazing family and a tight group of friends. She shined as a college student and as a leader in a local college ministry. She had been excited to enter the field of work she had been studying for, but then she experienced rejection after rejection. She had gotten to such a point of discouragement that she didn't want to be here anymore, and no one knew.

I followed up with her one-on-one, asking how she had gotten to such a place of despair and hadn't invited anyone in. She said she thought she had to be "strong." I asked where she had gotten her definition of strength. The next thing I knew, she was talking about her grandfather's funeral, where she and her family took up the front pew of the church. This young woman was crying her eyes out in grief. Then she looked down the row at her grandmother, the matriarch of the family. She was poised, unmoved, showing no emotion. "My grandmother was strong for everyone," she said. "And I guess when I think of strength, I think of my grandma."

Like her, you and I have had experiences that taught us how to handle grief, sadness, and pain. This young woman was invited to look strong even if she didn't feel strong. She was invited to avoid looking weak or emotional. And we get her. We get her because we too have been invited to be anything but hurt, anything but messy, anything but sad. Even if it means being anything but ourselves.

A woman who had just received a potential cancer diagnosis asked to meet with me because she was afraid to face hell *and* heaven. "Most of us are afraid of death and the idea of hell," I told her. "But tell me why you're afraid of heaven."

She said, "I am afraid to meet God."

When I probed, she said, "Well, I used to be involved in church, and now I'm not at all. I used to go to youth group multiple times a week, and now I never talk to God. A man used to tell me when he hurt me that it was all my fault and that I should be ashamed and pray to God to keep quiet. I have never understood the Bible and don't feel connected to it. I used to have so many friends at church, but I haven't been in so long, and I don't even take my kids. I used to, but sporadically. I don't feel God when I pray, so I just kind of stopped praying. Plus, I . . ."

"Whoa. Whoa. Whoa." I had to stop her. "We have to go back to something you said a few minutes ago. Are you saying that someone abused you as a child, and they made you believe that *God not only thought you deserved the abuse but that He was in on the secret*?"

Quiet like she was told to be, she nodded yes.

I was beyond upset. She had been taught to put up with the pain because God was in on it. With absolute certainty, I said, "If God is a God who wants you to be abused, to keep quiet, to feel ashamed like it's your fault, I don't want to go to heaven either. But that's not God! The God I know would never want you to be abused. He would never want you to suffer in silence. God would never want you to take on this shame as though you asked for it."

I knew that contrary to what this outrageous, abusive, horrific collision from hell had told her, God wanted to heal her, not harm her. I kept going: "What if Jesus is *not* who your wounds and *wounders* made Him out to be? What if when you meet God in heaven, there will be no more tears, no more abuse, no more sickness, no more goodbyes? I believe that it's not a place to fear, but a place of safety. And when you get there—because you will—you will overcome this terrible pain and its awful, awful lie. God will meet you, now and on the other side, with the most perfect, pure, unconditional love you can ever know."

The more I sit with women in their pain, the more sure I am that each one of us has been schooled in how to deal with pain and that many of the things we've learned cause us even more pain.

I wonder if what you and I were taught is serving us. Is the way you were shown to handle pain and hardship working? Are you healthy? Are you healed? Or are you still silent? Still pretending? Still trying to be strong for everyone else? Are you like me, still striving to be that good little girl, handling pain just like the hurting people in your life told you to?

My mother gave me up when I was fifteen, and that day she knocked on my door, we had not been in close geographic proximity for years. I liked it that way. I *wanted* it that way. I knew I could unlock the dead bolt and fake a welcome. I could open that door and offer her lemonade and a chance to hold her granddaughter. But nothing in me wanted to do that. So I had stayed in that closet, trying to keep my baby quiet, trying not to move, trying to keep my mother's life out of mine.

The knocks stopped for a moment. I didn't feel safe yet, so I pulled Bella close and held her tight so she would feel safe. "You're OK. Shhhhhhhh," I said, teaching my daughter to stay quiet, just like my mother taught me.

3

we don't move on

I spent most of my childhood hoping Mom would come home.

Nights were the hardest. During the day I'd go to school, and then I'd gallivant around in the afternoons. I'd play all day in the summers, hoping they could last forever. We town kids also went to the candy store, rode bikes, and came home when the siren wailed. Every night the siren sounded from the fire station at nine o'clock sharp. It trumpeted from ridge to ridge—a moment to recenter our entire town. Everyone knew what time it was. It set a rhythm and a cadence to our day and our night. All of us kids knew we had to be home when it beckoned. And all the parents knew they should be home too.

But sometimes parents don't do what they are told.

Mondays were the worst. They were Mom's day off from the café she owned. She'd party most of Sunday and wake up partying on Monday. By the time school got out, things were usually pretty ugly. Walking home, I would get this knot in the pit of my stomach, and I still get it now as a full-fledged adult. My mind would race and play out all the possible scenarios waiting for me. I prepared myself for every hypothetical. If this, then that. If she was running errands, then I would go play with friends. If she was at home but not in a state I liked keeping company with, I would have an avoidance tactic at the ready. If she wasn't home, I would search for her in hopes of controlling the outcome of our evening.

I would call the bars. I knew all their numbers by heart. I'd call the Brick Saloon, then the Pastime, then the Eagles Club, and if I got really desperate, I'd try the Old #3. I'd ask the bartender if Kim was there. I'd anxiously touch each number on the phone's number pad, counting to one hundred. If my mom hopped on the call, I'd yell at her like I was the demanding parent insisting on her presence. But no amount of anger, crying, or phone throwing made her come home when I wanted her to.

So I sat.

Alone.

Wishing not to be.

One . . . two . . . three . . . four . . . five . . . six . . . . . . one hundred.

My insides wailed long past the siren.

On nights Mom wasn't home and wasn't at work, there was a chance she was out having a good time. To be fair, this town had more bars per capita than any town I have ever been to. Sometimes I would skip the phone calls and go knocking at all the local establishments to find her. The old men would yell her name throughout the bar, like roll call in school, to see if she was in attendance. I would wait by the cracked-open door and peek in looking for her, hoping she wasn't there. I hoped she was at the grocery store or somewhere that wasn't going to end up with me waiting, alone, for who knows what.

When I found her, she would sometimes hand me a bag of Beer Nuts and tell me she would be home in a while. Beer Nuts were good, but they were never what I wanted.

The absence, the all-aloneness, ached. Loneliness said there was something about me that left me deservedly lonesome. Loneliness still finds me. And maybe loneliness finds you too. My loneliness was caused by someone else's loneliness, and maybe yours was as well. Loneliness is like a contagion. It spreads, orphaning daughters while their mothers go in search of a cure. We can feel like widows to our spouses' successes, loners to our loved ones' addictions, while the people we're supposed to be with go searching for something to make all that pain go away.

The very, very worst is loving someone with all the love you have yet seeing them hurt so deeply that their hurt starts hurting you too.

I tell my own kids I love them probably more than I should. I tell them almost to the point that they might be becoming calloused to the idea. I kiss them and hug them and love on them all day, every day. I think I get that from my mom. She always told me she loved me.

Mom had her good days when she wasn't drinking. She hugged me and spent time with me and took me on wild vacations. Life was always an adventure with her. We road-tripped in a school bus to the great state of Texas. We drove hours and hours to hit up foodie joints that were all the rage. She would savor the flavors and describe for me what was in each bite. "That has a bit of nutmeg," she would guess. Or, "You can taste the saffron," she might say. She taught me that the best secret ingredient to any sandwich is cilantro pesto mayo and to always use my steak leftovers to make a mean beef Stroganoff.

She carted me to all the Bob Dylan concerts she could. She took me on café errands and taught me how to take orders, ring up customers, and close up the tips at the end of the night. We set up camp near Cooper Lake for a month at a time in the summers, making baked beans on the fire, swimming with our dogs, and playing canoe tag on the lake at dark. She listened to me make speeches about Martin Luther King Jr., and she would applaud and say, "You're such a neat kid."

My mom really loved me.

Perhaps the most agonizing pain is when someone loves you, but you aren't enough, even so. You aren't enough to hold things together. You aren't enough to quit for. You aren't enough for them to change. You aren't enough to keep the people who are supposed to love you close by.

You aren't enough to come home for when the siren wails.

You not being enough becomes your truth. And this "truth" begins to lie to you, and when it does, you can no longer see yourself for who you truly are or see the people around you for who they truly are. My mom loved me, but that didn't always draw her home. And those nights alone began to speak to me in ways that cut deeper than I ever knew.

I knew I was loved. But I was also sure I wasn't enough.

Some days, if I got real scared or anxious about what Mom might bring home, I would run to my Aunt Jill's house. There, I knew what to expect at every visit. I loved sitting on the stone wall in her garden, soaking in the sunshine, surrounded by orange and yellow nasturtiums. I loved eating her sugar snap peas right off the vine. I loved her old-school bathtub with all sorts of scented lotions and potions. I loved that Jill was home at night. I loved having my cousin Andrea as a playmate and wondered if this might be what having a sibling was like. The two of us loved to play pretend "café."

Mom owned a hip little eatery that probably birthed the first hipsters, who didn't even know they were hip. Vegans could get a really good veggie burger before they knew they were vegans. Mom pesto'd, pickle'd, and aioli'd in the '80s. Her way with food was so magical, people drove hours from Seattle to our small town of Roslyn to eat her delicacies.

The food was incredible. It was homemade because there is no other way. The peanut butter pie was to die for, and so were the beef tips with béarnaise and the chicken breasts stuffed with spinach cream sauce. I didn't grow up asking, "What's for dinner?" I grew up ordering off a divine menu. The café was my living room.

I was at my aunt's once, enjoying my time as usual. Andrea was always the waitress and the cook, and I was always the customer. She would make a menu, but we both knew she didn't really have turkey tetrazzini or chicken cordon bleu. We knew that I had to order the same thing every time. Andrea would bring me water and then give me time to "think about" what I wanted. Every time I ordered, I would say with the confidence of a regular, "I'll take the peanut butter balls." Then Andrea would whip up the best everything-but-the-kitchen-sink balls with coconut and honey and nuts and whatever else she could find, and I would rave about how good they were.

That day, just like always, I was pretending to leave her the biggest tip, with honey all over my fingers, when pandemonium set in right outside our "restaurant."

Mom had driven her car through the neighbor's yard.

A good day, followed by a good day, followed by a good day, followed by a hellish day, followed by a good day. That was what was on my menu. I wasn't just a regular at Andrea's café, I was a regular to this way of Mom's life, ordering up the same thing again and again, even if I didn't want to.

I wonder what someone else's life ordered up for you. What message has wailed loudly in your life for far too long? What does it say, and how does it still scream at you? I wonder what world you tried escaping with pretend and what you were expected to endure.

I don't think most of us quite understand the amount of courage it takes to leave your life and flee for safety. After my incredibly strong mother got us out of that incredibly frightening nightmare with John years ago, we didn't look back. We moved into the first rental we could find until Mom bought a house a block or so away from her café.

I had a purple room, which was way cool for a middle schooler, and we had orange-painted floors and a ceramic smoking frog that puffed on hand-rolled cigarettes and blew smoke rings. You had one too, *riiiight*?

Our new place brought hope of a new start.

One morning in middle school, I popped out of bed, peeked in to see if my mom had come home the night before, ate some Grape-Nuts, and got ready for school. I tried teasing my bangs to rock 1985, and because my mom was asleep, I sneaked the forbidden eyeliner, grabbed my backpack, and headed out. I got about four steps down our front porch and was confronted by a frenzy. A bunch of men from town were trying to get a car back up over the edge of a bluff in front of our house. As the neighbors pulled the rope with all their might, the car began to appear. I was sick. With recognition. It was *myyyy mommmm's* car.

I sped up, trying to get away from this drunk-driving scene without anyone seeing me.

Not only was I panicking, I was mortified. I mean, starting your period in public in middle school is embarrassing, and so is not getting asked to slow dance at the social. But this? This wasn't something you could graduate from. This way of life always left *me* with the hangover of her drunken stupors. And that wasn't going away the next week or the next year or maybe ever. I ran as fast as I could away from all that I had no control over, to walk into what I *could* control.

At school, I could morph letters and create stories with words. I could do my darndest to capture boys' attention. I could work hard to look prettier. I could practice and practice and practice basketball to land starting guard. I could enter the popularity contest and try my best to win. I could attempt to charm Mr. Butkovich, my grumpy social studies teacher, and even sometimes get him to smile. But no amount of trying to control one of my worlds changed the other.

First period bell rang, and I filed my mom's car-over-the-edge-of-an-embankment in my Pee-Chee folder along with my book report on *The Diary of Anne Frank*. We could all hide for safety.

My mom and I never did talk about why her car was over the side of a hill. Instead, I came home from school, and we ate beet borscht and watched *Entertainment Tonight*.

Mom always asked me to move on without asking me.

But I didn't move on. I moved *with*. All the pain, it moved with me every single day. It moved into my teens, my twenties, and my thirties. It became my story, my baggage, my reason for squatting in a freaking closet.

Friend, in case no one's told you, we don't move on. We move *with*.

Home alone, lying in my bed one windy night, I could hear the screen door creak. It took a lot of effort to climb into my bed. I would step onto the window seat and climb a ladder to my loft bed that left a few feet between my face and the ceiling. I used to shave my legs up there in the dark because Mom had forbidden it. She wanted me to go free and natural and not care about what I looked like. But as a middle schooler, I did care about what I looked like. So I shaved in secret. Sometimes I would cut my entire shin, but the risk was worth it. I might get grounded. I might injure myself. But I wouldn't have hairy legs!

I heard noises outside the bathroom window, which was next to my bedroom. *It could be a stray cat or a broken screen*, I reassured myself. But the commotion moved from the outside of the house to the inside. Someone was breaking in. It was him.

The man who had taken his rage out on us had broken into our new place.

What could I do? I didn't have a phone or a weapon or a dad. I mean, I had a dad, but who knows where he was or what he was doing. All I knew was that he was never around when I needed a dad most. I lay there, scared stiff.

I heard him grumbling as he paced from the bathroom to the kitchen, to the living room, to Mom's room, and then back to the dining room. He couldn't find her. I pretended to be asleep.

John dragged one of the orange-painted dining room chairs across the floor, sat down, and waited for her to come home.

I couldn't breathe. Fear takes your breath away. It paralyzes you. Fear didn't move on. It moved in. And when fear moves in, it becomes a part of you, always, *always*, waiting for what might be next.

The fear I felt that night was never discussed, never calmed. The same waiting for what is about to come, that same kind of agony, can find me on any ordinary day in any ordinary place even now. It can find me irrationally, and it can find me at peace. It finds me when I'm anxious about my kids. It finds me in circumstances that feel out of my control. It finds me living in hypotheticals, overanalyzing, acting on assumptions, being overprotective, feeling insecure, and becoming frenzied with worry. I can get scared in a bathroom stall, in my own bedroom, on an airplane, and at a book club full of moms.

Once fear moves in, it's almost as hard to evict as an enraged man in love with the woman his anger lost.

I was speaking at a women's retreat when I met a woman who couldn't stop tripping over her emotions. Throughout the weekend, she kept wanting to talk about why she was not fine but also wanting to tell me she was *totally fine*. At one point she said, "Shouldn't I be over this since it was more than a decade ago? I mean, if I'm good with God, why am I still crying?"

She had bought into a theology that said not only that her permission to cry or grieve had expired but that she should not be sad if she had a Savior. She was trying to assure me that she had a happy present but didn't understand why she was still crying about a sad past. I had to ask, "Did someone tell you that as a Christian, you should pick yourself up by the bootstraps, move on, and not be sad about sad things?"

"Yes . . ." she said. "Yes, they did."

There was clearly something she wasn't over, as much as she tried to pretend she was, so I asked, "What haaaappppened ten years ago?"

She explained. She had almost married a guy she had been dating, but after coming to the realization that they were headed in different directions and didn't share faith, she had broken up with him.

And then he committed suicide.

Her spiritual mentors tried scurrying her past her grief by saying things like "You did the right thing" and "There's no need to be sad when you have Jesus." They wanted her to be "fine." But she hadn't been fine. And here she was years later, still trying to pretend she was. I couldn't help but blurt out, "Of course you are still sad! Someone ending their life is tragic!"

This woman's emotions were telling her she needed to make room to grieve the loss of a love and a loved one. They were telling her, "You are still crying because you still hurt." Perhaps the same is true for you. You are still sad because you're still sad. You are still angry because you're still angry. You're still shut down because you're still shut down.

There was no room for sadness, guilt, or tears for this woman. She was not invited to grieve but instead asked to giddyup and get on with it. But we don't often just move on without being affected, do we?

Did you try to move on from something painful but find that it still moves with you? Were you expected to be unaffected by an anxiety-inducing experience? Is the mess you were asked to overlook still messing with you? Is the sting from a friend still stinging? Are the names they called you still naming you? Is the denial you were asked to accommodate stealing your truth? Is the addiction you were asked to normalize still haunting you years later? Is the abuse you were asked to keep quiet still screaming at you? Is the siren still wailing that when you are alone, you deserve to be?

Unless we have experienced *actual healing*, we don't move on. We move *with*. We move with the cutting pain, the unrelenting fear, the pervasive anxiety, the damaging habits, the lingering emotions, and the unresolved trauma.

I moved with my pain right into a closet, holding Bella. We were still so tightly squeezed in that tiny closet space that the hangers started making a ruckus. I was sweating, surrounded by winter coats and luggage, trying to soothe my daughter. I found myself having an angry hypothetical conversation, like one does, where I was actually being honest with my mother: *You can't just show up at my door and expect me to "move on," expect me to forget, expect me to eat your beet borscht. You never owned any of your mess, and you made so much of it. You just expected me to embrace it, and I did. I embraced* your *mess . . .*

And now I *am one.*

4

not dealing is not healing

(and Ten Other Wounded Ways We Try to Heal)

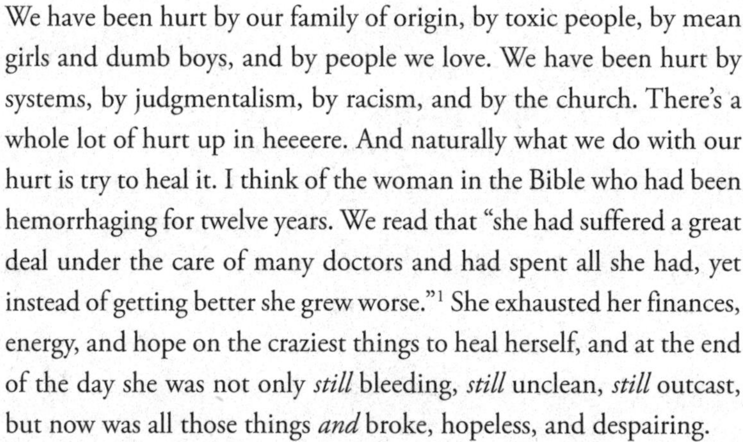

We have been hurt by our family of origin, by toxic people, by mean girls and dumb boys, and by people we love. We have been hurt by systems, by judgmentalism, by racism, and by the church. There's a whole lot of hurt up in heeeere. And naturally what we do with our hurt is try to heal it. I think of the woman in the Bible who had been hemorrhaging for twelve years. We read that "she had suffered a great deal under the care of many doctors and had spent all she had, yet instead of getting better she grew worse."[1] She exhausted her finances, energy, and hope on the craziest things to heal herself, and at the end of the day she was not only *still* bleeding, *still* unclean, *still* outcast, but now was all those things *and* broke, hopeless, and despairing.

Like this woman, we instinctively try to heal ourselves, and I think it's partly because we were intended to be whole. When we aren't, when we feel broken, we go seeking a solution, a cure. But what I've learned is that half the things we try end up hurting us even more.

There are a million wounded ways we try to heal ourselves, but let's talk about ten of them.

We "*spend all we have trying.*" Apparently in those days, it was thought that there were eleven ways to cure the bleeding woman's kind of sickness. And they were weird, like "carrying the ashes of an ostrich egg in a linen rag in summer and a cotton rag in winter."[2] My guess is she tried every one of them, because that's what we do when we get desperate for change. We think "if I just" get a man, go to a naturopath, lose twenty pounds, snarf down spinach, apply essential oils to my earlobes, and pray with bigger words . . . We will try everything before we try Jesus. We will even try the keto diet before we try God. And often all the things we try leave us still in need of healing.

We *God over it.* Some people beer over it. A lot of Christians try to get over it by overspiritualizing their pain. They try to slap Jesus on it and call it good. You know we do this, because you have experienced people doing it for you. When you are awkwardly crying and people are uncomfortable, they are quick to say, "Let me pray for you." Now don't get me wrong, prayer is awesome. But sometimes it is used to end the discomfort someone is feeling because the emotions are too much. We've also had well-intentioned friends God-smack us with a statement they hope will fast-forward us straight to happy. They say, "You have Jesus, so you don't need to despair." Or, "This too shall pass. God will use your pain for His glory." And while that might be true, it invites us to minimize our suffering and skip the "needs healing" part. It tells us to get right to the "I'm good 'cause I have God" part. This leaves us hurting, in need of healing, and not going to God or God's people for help, because every time we do, we feel like it's *Jesus* dismissing our pain, which really hurts. We know this God-overing-it won't work, but we keep trying because that's what good little Christians do.

We also try to heal by *numbing*. We turn to cheap fixes to self-medicate. What do you think you're doing when you binge-watch *Ted Lasso*? You're trying to escape into a story that's not your own. What do you think you're doing when you want to drink red wine every night? If you're like me, you're wanting to take the edge off, to not feel, to ease your own reality. We numb with overworking, doomscrolling, online shopping, porn, overeating, exercise obsession, weed, self-harm, sarcasm, procrastination, success highs, overchurching, and more. The issue is that most of us are self-medicating to the point that the things we use to numb our pain are wounding us even more. We need to feel to heal. Feeling helps us find clarity on what hurts. When we avoid feeling, we are in effect taking away the God-given indicators we need to experience so that we know we are hemorrhaging and in need of help.

Another wounded way we try to heal is by *acting like it never hurt*. When a memory surfaces, we make it small. We minimize the sting of someone's words, someone's betrayal, someone's toxicity. We act like it wasn't a big deal, like it didn't bother us. We do this because often that's what the people who hurt us did. They wounded us, and then they said, "You're fine, stop your whining." They ridiculed us publicly and then said, "What are you gonna do? Cryyyy?" They put a Band-Aid on our owies and expected us to stop talking about it. So that's what we are still doing. We are dismissing our own pain, so it never finds a remedy. You can't heal a hurt you can't name.

We also *justify sick behavior*. We say, "They didn't know better," almost as though that makes it hurt less. We say, "They meant well," as though their intentions disregard the pain of their actions. We say, "They came from a hard family upbringing," to excuse the baggage we now carry because they handed it to us. If we justify sick behavior, then we don't have to say, "This actually happened, and it was really wrong. It was harmful. Traumatic." As long as we keep making excuses for hurtful people, we get to fend off our own need for healing from the hurt they caused. And of course we do that because we love to run and hide from our own pain.

We *blame-shift*. What will make us feel better about our dad not showing up for us? Blame our stepmom. What will make us feel better about our pastor being manipulative? Blame God. What will make us feel better about the pain *we* caused? Blame the person we hurt for triggering our anger. We do a lot of blame-shifting to try to feel better, but it never actually heals.

We *self-protect to the point of injury*. Some of us have been soooo hurt, so what do we do? We try to protect our lives in such a way that no one else can hurt us. This leads to isolation, disconnection, unhealthy relationships, overcontrolling, growth avoidance, stunted emotions, fear of vulnerability, perfectionism, trust issues, and much more. Our attempts to self-protect often hurt more than help.

We *run from ourselves*. We stay so busy, so scheduled, so amped up on activity that we never actually have to think, feel, or look in the mirror. If we're busy enough, we don't have to deal with what's really going on. A friend once told me she couldn't be alone. I had this sense in my gut that she was running from something she didn't want to face. It turns out she had been having an affair for over a year, and being alone meant she would have to feel and deal with all the reasons she found herself there. Our crazy calendars are often the way we unknowingly schedule "not dealing."

Some of us try to *prove our worth* to take away the pain. We spend years trying to prove to the people who hurt us that we are awesome, that their wounds do not hold power over our lives, that we are untouchable. I have a friend, a very successful friend, who has spent her entire life building an empire because so many people told her she wasn't enough. She still hasn't healed, but she lets that hurt drive her hustle. And yes, there's something to be said about purposing our pain, but we also have to *deal with* that pain. We have to recognize that we might still hurt and we might still need healing because no matter how successful we get, our achievements don't make the pain go away.

We also *hide our mess* hoping that if we look good, we'll feel good. It's like we are our closets in middle school. Remember that? Mom said, "Clean your room!" So what did we do? We threw all the mess in the closet and the room was clean! But it wasn't clean. It looked like it was, but it was in utter disarray, and if our mom had opened the closet door, it would all have come crashing out onto the floor—the training bras, chip bags, hair scrunchies, mixtapes, and "Dear diary, I love so-and-so's." We are like middle school closets. Our "room" is clean because no one sees our resentment, our anger, our insecurities. But the mess—it's in there. And it's sure to embarrassingly spill out as soon as someone tries to open the door.

Here's the deal: Pain that we don't deal with comes out sideways! We think we can stuff it inside, ignore it, cover it, or hide it, but it comes out in ways we don't want it to. It comes out in passive-aggressive comments at family gatherings. It comes out in hatred and unforgiveness. It comes out in panic attacks. Sometimes, it comes out in stomachaches, or in lashing out at your kids, or in unhealthy habits that you use to soothe yourself. Unhealed pain always comes out sideways, and if you're like me, you'll find yourself running and hiding from it, and then it will decide to stage an unwanted intervention on your life.

Here is what I know for sure, friend: Not dealing is not healing. So maybe, here together, we can start to deal, so we can start to heal.

5

a wounded collision

Within a week of hiding in that closet with my baby, I went and surprised you and found myself sitting across from a therapist. As you'd predict, the first thing she asked was, "What brings you in today?"

I answered with sarcasm, "I'm here because I'm playing hide-and-seek. By myself." I laughed, but we both knew my humor couldn't mask my issues.

I had given my messy, broken life to Jesus ten years prior and spent the last decade running into Him and experiencing His transformation. But it became so glaringly obvious in that closet that I needed more healing.

I explained what led to the hide-and-seek, which was my mother's sudden move back into my everyday life after ditching me at age fifteen. Here she was, standing on my doorstep, wanting to be a part of the family I had worked so hard to make safe and healthy and stable.

Ever since I was a teenager, my mother and I had managed to have minimal, short visits, but to now have her do daily life with me?

That was too much. For years Mom had been living in Hawaii, and I, in Washington. The truth is, the distance between us was far greater than the Pacific Ocean that separated us, and I liked it that way.

I tried to explain my history with my mother to this counselor. She abruptly jumped to, "You need to severely limit the time you spend with your mom. Keep it to thirty minutes a week."

Thirty minutes? That's not nearly enough . . . and . . . it's way too much.

It's always been Mom and me. No husband, no stepdad, no boyfriend—not one stuck. No brother, no sister, no sibling—not one kept. But Mom kept me. She took me to a Bob Dylan concert when I was a week old and baptized me. Of course, I wasn't actually baptized, but the fact that Mom *says* I was tells you a lot. In his song "Property of Jesus," Dylan sings, "You've picked up quite a story and you've changed since the womb. What happened to the real you, you've been captured but by whom?"[1]

To answer his question, the real me never had a chance to be. My story picked up my mother's. I was born into her groans, pain, and pushing. I was born into her crazy, her genius, her ache. I was born into her wild, her whimsy, her weird.

I inherited her poverty as a protest and her protest as a principle.

I was changed by her hairbrained ideas, her hippie wandering, her stubborn and unruly desire to be self-dependent, her addiction, picking these up as though they were mine too.

The moment I breathed this polluted air and breastfed for sustenance, I needed her. I needed her to be my mother, and I needed her to be my father. I needed her to be my protector, my peace, my provider.

I needed her to be my teacher and my guide. And she needed me too. I could be her cure.

As I was growing up, if Mom felt pain, I felt pain. If she was stressed, I carried that stress. If Mom needed a cover, I covered for her. If she was sad, I felt sad. When Mom was tired, I would massage her back and spell out a message on her skin that she would have to guess. With my pointer finger I would inscribe as clearly as possible . . .

I L O V E Y O U

I'd wait to see if she could guess.

She always did.

"I love you too," she would say.

One night she woke me up out of a deep sleep, frantic and with blood all over her face. She had run her car into a telephone pole down the street. She needed help, and though I had no idea how to help, I did my best. I got towels and hot water and wiped off the blood, whipping out my grown-up first aid skills as a ten-year-old. She did the same for me when I was sick, sad, or hurting.

No one asked me to, but I made it my job to take on my mom's pain. It was my responsibility to bring her relief. When she sat on the floor drunk, sad about what was happening in the world, I would sit on the floor and get sad too. When Mom was stressed over doing the café books and cabernet and Ella Fitzgerald weren't enough, I tried stand-up comedy. When she was laughing, I was laughing. When she was despairing, I was despairing. I got up in the night when she needed a friend. I understood loneliness too.

Our *we* was all we had. And our *we* needed more than *us*.

We were intertwined, perhaps so connected, so braided, that it was beautiful and dangerous. Our *we* had a bond so strong, a love so fierce, and an understanding that spoke its own language. Our *we* also had a weight no child should ever have to bear. Maybe you know all too well the heaviness of carrying a weight you never should have?

Years of bitterness and distrust found me wanting to agree with the counselor's advice. She was right. I should limit my mom's presence like some kind of consequence. I should tell her what an ugly drunk she was. I should recount the ways she had hurt me. I should make a list of all the ways she couldn't get her act together to save us. I figured it was my turn. I should be able to not get *my* act together for once. I should send *her* packing like she sent me. I should tell her about the countdown clock that ticks away those thirty minutes in great expectation of when we won't be together. 30 . . . 29 . . . 28 . . . 27 . . .

A-*freaking*-men. Finally I could feel free from this relationship. I could say, "Enough is enough. I am sick and tired of dealing with your issues, lady." Finally, I could be released of the burden I have carried my whole life, and it could be counselor approved.

Mom carried me on her back while she picked apples in the gorgeous Okanogan Country to pay the rent. We lived in a hippie commune in Seattle with other single moms who all shared breastfeeding, cooking, bills, and childcare, creating the village they needed but didn't have. Mom and I lived in a school bus, traveled Indonesia, and campaigned for Jesse Jackson together. My mother taught me to play checkers, dominoes, and cribbage. She also showed me how to make a mean manicotti, a good cheese sauce, and a delicious pasta on the fly.

When I was around three, we moved into an old historic building in an old historic town. She had enough passion and foolishness to pull off turning this old brothel into a popular café that people traveled to, from far and wide, to feel loved and full.

Mom was different from other moms. She toted a stuffed animal that she had cut open and made a purse out of. She smoked Camel cigarettes and refused to stand for "The Star-Spangled Banner" at my school sporting events. She didn't care about fitting in. She lived with a rebellious spirit that questioned the status quo, an adventurous spirit that made even the mundane wacky and fun, and an open spirit that collected all sorts of crazy characters along the way. She always saw the magnificence of color, the beauty of race, and the richness of diversity. Your money wouldn't impress her, neither would your title. Your amazing jazz album collection might. And a good cheese—that would do the trick too.

There was an old jukebox in the café that lit the place up and bebopped tunes that took people to places and times they longed for. We had live jazz bands and belly dancers and theme nights. In a very small town where a common complaint was lack of things to do, Mom created a place where there was always something going on. This village she fostered was hip and cool, attracting people from all walks of life. There were loggers dining with tree huggers, Republicans drinking Bloody Marys with Democrats, and hippies feasting with rednecks. And I wouldn't have had it any other way.

Mom wasn't just a drunk. It would have been easier if she was. I could have closed that door she knocked on and kept that thing closed. But she was so much more. Yes, she would often end the week drinking for several days straight, but before that, she worked hard at the things that were important to her. Mom was strong in her convictions about materialism and the environment and racial reconciliation. She fought for civil rights and women's rights and rights for just about anyone whose rights had been taken away.

Mom came in clutch for things that needed saving. She hired people that no one else would give a chance. I swear, she gave all her boyfriends jobs. She fought for trees like some people fight for family, and she took in people who needed a place to belong. Mom was really good at handing out belonging.

She lived with the orthodoxy of a priest without the religion, called to serve the earth and its resources. She reused her ziplock bags. She saved whales and volunteered with environmental organizations.

She started a business called the Leftover Queen because she could make a delectable soup out of any leftovers in your fridge or mine. She could take your jar of capers, your Dijon mustard, and your days-old basmati rice and turn it into something you wish you could eat every day. But you will never eat it again because she didn't use recipes.

Some people say they value quality time. My mom valued time together so much that her gifts to others always included an experience: camel riding, train tripping, skiing, thrifting, art making, silly hat wearing, animal sanctuary visiting, or Japanese taiko concert-going. Presence is what she gave and what she hoped to receive.

How could I . . . abandon my mother? Thirty minutes? The bond we shared, the love we felt, the life we'd experienced, and the understanding we had, all rebelled against that thirty-minute timer. But the abuse we'd suffered, the loneliness I'd endured, the secrets I kept . . . All my pain wanted that limit.

My feelings fought each other in a no-win battle. I didn't know how to protect myself without hurting my mom. My love and loyalty to her fought my hatred and bitterness, and that exhausted me. Every single time I was with her, she dismissed our past, and that brought pain to our present.

Part of me couldn't pretend anymore, and part of me wanted to. I'd been pretending for years. She taught me to. I was an actor in her play, going along with the story the way she told it. You're right, Mom. Alcohol is not the problem. I'm the problem. Let's just keep pretending that everything that happened didn't happen. Let's never talk about it. Let's just blame everything else but what's really to blame.

In our time apart, I had done years of hard soul work. I now had a family culture that my husband and I created intentionally. We value full authenticity and no make-believe. But my mom didn't know how to live that way. And here she was, back on my scene, trying to roll in and be Super Grandma, which would require me to be super fake.

Pretending would hurt me, but the truth would hurt her. If I was honest with her, she would drink to numb the pain my honesty caused. And drinking more would only cause her—and me—more suffering. This was the double bind I lived with constantly. I wanted to run as far away as I could. I wanted the Pacific Ocean between us again.

A part of me wanted to agree with the counselor, and a part of me wanted to protect my mom. Another part of me wanted to escape the reality of this being my life. And all of me was fighting to find what God wanted from me outside the closet.

In the midst of battling these opposing feelings, it was like *another* Person walked into the counseling office. I don't know if I have ever experienced such a strong Presence in a room before. It was like *theeee* Counselor showed up. Suddenly everything in me revolted against what the therapist advised. Like a crazy psycho mom who hides in closets with babies, I blurted, "Noooooooo!"

It was dead quiet.

I don't think the *lowercase* counselor was expecting that response from a nice chick like me. I am usually more receptive to counsel. It wasn't that I think boundaries are a bad idea or that they are not often absolutely necessary. In fact, I have held boundaries with my mom in the past. But I knew God was asking for something more this time.

Setting a timer on my mother would have been a justification to keep running, keep escaping, keep pretending. None of that was healing me, and none of that was healing her.

"What will that accomplish?! How will that heal?" I cried out to the walls, to the therapist, to the hurt that needed an actual remedy.

Would my thirty minutes undo the years of her pain that led to mine? Will avoidance make all my pain and yours go away? Will building more walls repair all our brokenness, or will refusal to forgive bring reconciliation? Can we find the peace we long for by pushing away the people who hurt us? Is our fake "I have to pretend I like the people I am called to love" working to build actual close, healthy relationships?

In that office, my heart was breaking. I was overwhelmingly grieved for all this brokenness: my brokenness, your brokenness, and the brokenness of the ones who hurt us. My strong response came from outside of me. And it was so intense, it shut down niceties. It changed everything in me from that day forward. What came out of my mouth, I had never heard, thought, or felt before. It was like, with each word uttered, I realized its truth:

"I was . . . I was born into wounds.

"I collided with wounds that wounded me.

"*My parents* were hurt.

"They never got healing for their wounds, and then we collided and they wounded me . . . and I have been colliding with others and wounding them. It's all just one big . . .

". . . wounded collision."

This was *the* moment when I began to see not just who I am or where I was, but how I got here. How we *all* got here.

I saw my mom as that blonde, blue-eyed little girl on skis, ready to take on the mountain, just like the picture of her I keep in my Bible, pocketed in Isaiah 53. I saw her watching *her* mom drown loneliness in cocktail parties and social hours. I saw her longing to be close to a dad who was distant, private, and busy. I saw that smart, fun, adventurous little girl growing into a woman who had suffered the agony of watching her mother drink herself to death. And I saw the little girl in me watching the little girl in her take drink after drink after drink to numb all her sorrow. And every sip that numbed my mother's wounds birthed *mine*.

In this room with two counselors, I saw the pain that never got healing hurt me. And I also saw that if my pain didn't get healing, I would hurt my little girl.

This is true for all of us. We have all collided with wounded people who never got healing. And their hurt, hurt us. All that heartache we feel—all that bruising, fear, and insecurity, all the self-medicating, tears, and bitterness, all the ways we feel held back, messy, and damaged—most of it was procured by someone's pain that was caused by someone else's pain that was caused by someone else's pain. Imagine if their pain had been healed before it hurt us. Imagine how different you and I would be. Now our wounds have the great, great capacity to wound everyone we collide with, including our own kids.

Wounds unhealed continue to wound and wound, because wounded people wound people. When I understood this, I began to see those who had wounded me not as people who deserve my anger, my distance, my walls, but as people who need *the very same thing I do*.

Healing.

I realized I wanted for my mom what I wanted for myself. We both needed God. Our lives were begging for Him. And when you finally see that you need the very same thing the person who wounded you does, it changes something. Somehow you were both wronged and abandoned. You were both thirsty and numbing, lost and searching, both wanting what you were intended to have but never got. You were both just two people who collided with someone else's wounds.

I knew from years of running into Jesus that when He collides with wounded people, they are left more whole than broken. But not so with us. Our collisions with others often seem to leave us more battered and more broken. When I collide with hurting people, I hurt back, I run, I hide in closets. I needed Jesus to enter my pain, not leave me alone in it. I needed Jesus to stand in my mess, not ditch me until it was cleaned up. I knew that what I needed for my own healing was what my mother needed for hers.

I started crying as I processed out loud.

"I have got to, *got to*, fiiiigure ouuuut how to love the person who wounded me the most. That's what Jesus does."

It had taken ten years of collision after collision, running into Jesus, to be able to say those words. I finally understood that God doesn't run from pain—mine or anyone else's. God was calling me to no longer push my hurting mother away nor pretend I didn't hurt. He was calling me to heal. Maybe my healing and your healing are the only chance we have to stop all this pain from traveling from one collision to the next, one generation to the next. I couldn't shake the invitation—and maybe absolute charge—God was handing me, to follow Him into pain rather than run from it. My yearning became a desire not only for my own healing, but for *her* healing and *your* healing.

I mean, don't you want it? Aren't you tired of all this hurt? Aren't our lives begging for help and health and wholeness? Don't you want to be made well and see the people you love being made well? What if it's possible? What if the healing you long for is actually possible? Jesus says it is.

I gave the counselor lady her eighty-five bucks. She probably assumed I'd go home and keep playing hide-and-seek every time the doorbell rang. But what really happened was *theeee* Counselor said to me as I walked to my car: *You're going to do something with these two words . . .*

wounded
collision.

6

left more whole than broken

After I collided with Jesus in that counseling office, I began to view all of life—pain, sin, people, my mom, my dad, and even you and me—with completely new eyes. Those two words, "wounded collision," began to radically change the way I see the world. I now see we are *all* colliding, and if we are wounded, we wound each other.

This doesn't explain only dramatic and traumatic events, but it explains even those irritating run-ins we have with people who drive us nuts. Wounded collisions happen every day. This is what is happening when Ice Queen Snob Girl runs into you at book club. When your boss is on a power bender to let everyone know who's in control. When psycho Mr. and Mrs. Jones are trying to "win" by pitting their child against yours. And in a one-night stand when two people exchange sex but want love.

She is an ice queen because letting people in has never worked in her favor. Your boss is on a power trip because they are afraid people won't respect them unless they are in control and in charge. Mr. and Mrs. Jones are competing with your kids so they can be seen as "winners" because somewhere along the way they lost big-time. Those people you might call "slutty" are giving their bodies away for love because they believe they aren't worthy of love without giving something away to get it.

You are wounded, and you bump into their wounds. They are wounded, and they bump into your wounds.

Boom.

Wounded collision.

We need a new kind of collision! And from what I have seen and experienced in Jesus, He crashes right into our messy, wounded lives, and when He does, we are left more whole than broken. When we look at the life of Jesus in the New Testament, we see the outcast restored to community, the hemorrhaging woman healed, the woman bent over by a spirit set free. When Jesus ran into people, their shame was sent packing, their wounded views of others were healed, their need to drink from dirty wells was relieved.

That day in therapy, I wanted this change for my own life, but apparently God wanted it for more than just me. A week or two after I walked out of that counseling office, a college-aged student named Brittany asked if I would be her mentor. I'd just walked out of hiding in a closet with my baby, so I questioned if I was the mentoring type. Still, I suggested we get together and look at what happened in the New Testament when Jesus collided with wounded people. Brittany was excited about this idea—so excited that to my surprise, she showed up to my house with twenty friends!

These young women piled into my living room over the next few years, watching Jesus collide with hurting people in the Bible. We started noticing who He ran into: religious bullies, people with nasty skin rashes, girls who would sleep with your boyfriend, and people who would betray you on the fly. And He healed them! As we watched Him heal them, He was healing us. He was healing small things and big things, past things and present things.

When Jesus restored the man's shriveled hand, He also restored these college girls' shriveled self-esteems. When Jesus set free the woman caught in adultery, he also set free a girl in my living room who had been steeped in shame. Jesus was healing the way we viewed people and the way we viewed ourselves. He was healing our bitterness, our envy, and our insecurity. He was healing our distorted body image issues and our false ideas about what we have to do to be lovable. He was healing the lies we believed about ourselves, and He was healing the brokenness that got in the way of our relationships.

Fran, a young woman I was walking alongside, shared with me that her father had sexually abused her growing up. He said it was their "little secret," like what they had shared was this special thing. The more Fran ran into Jesus' pure and perfect love, the more she saw that the love she had known from her father was perverse and damaging. Fran began to trust Jesus with her story and her pain, her desire to be loved, and her hopes for healing. I watched her collide, and it changed her.

Our group ran into this beautiful Christ in all our brokenness, and I was leading these girls out of mine. As I was changing, they were changing, and as they were changing, I was changing. It was like nothing I had experienced before. There was something different, something unique, something God-touched that we experienced together in what those girls named the Wounded Collision Bible Study.

And then one of the girls was in an actual wounded collision—much worse, a deadly one. As Christine was on her way to work, a high school student rear-ended her car and sent it flying into a family in a crosswalk. Through no fault of her own, a young child was killed.

This was absolutely horrific for the family who lost their daughter, the high schooler whose distracted driving will forever imprint her life, and our dear friend Christine who was at the absolute worst place at the worst time. No amount of Christian answers could make this feel OK. For days, weeks, months, and years, our group walked alongside her. We needed Jesus to run into our pain more than ever. We didn't need Him just for our past pain but our present. We needed God to be with our friend as anxiety started paralyzing her decisions, her travels, and her dreams. And we watched Christine trust God, bravely say yes to counseling, begin to leave the house, get in a car again, be real about her grief, and let us carry her.

Over time, most of the girls graduated and moved away from our college town, but a few stuck around and wanted to keep meeting. God challenged us to step outside our group and invite more women in. So we tried an experiment and called it "Collide."

More than fifty college-aged girls came to our first event, and it was gloriously beautiful. We planned another one, and eighty showed up, and then we planned another, and another. At one point I looked up and saw a sanctuary full of hundreds of women of all ages, women with diverse life experiences, women from all different denominations, women who don't set foot in church, and a woman with a poodle in her purse. I about fell over. I ran upstairs where two college-aged guys, old students of mine, were running the sound booth. They had been helping all year, watching this experiment unfold. I put my hands on their shoulders. Breathing heavily, like the wind had been knocked out of me, I said, "Oh. My. Gosh. I think I'm in wiiiiiiiimen's ministry."

They looked at me like I'd lost my ever-loving mind. "You didn't know you were in women's ministry?!" they teased.

"Noooo! But there is a woman with a poodle in her purse downstairs, and I have to luuuuhv her."

I think the indelible moment when it hit me that God was creating something remarkable out of pain was when I ran into a woman after a Collide event. We had just ministered to hundreds of women, practically on accident. I was picking up trash when an older woman scurried between pews to catch me on the other side. She just stood there, so I introduced myself.

At first she couldn't speak, but then she muttered her name. Deeply emotional, she said something had struck her that day. She and her husband had been highly involved in the church. Her husband died, and then she lost her son to suicide. She said the church treated her horribly. They couldn't handle the topic. People either pitied her or told her that her son was in hell. That was when she stopped going to church. After that, she faced the attempted suicide of her daughter. She told me with no emotion whatsoever what she had told herself: "It's fine. I planned a funeral for my husband. I planned a funeral for my son. I can plan a funeral for my daughter."

This precious woman had experienced so much pain and wounding—and had been made to believe God couldn't handle it. And here, years later, she had walked through the doors of Collide, and we gave her permission to be broken before God. We promised her that He could handle it all. She collided with Jesus in her deep grief. Her heart had become like a stone to protect itself from breaking into a million pieces. In tears and anguish, she said, "I didn't allow myself to feel, and today I feel." It hurts to feel. But we are made to feel. It is there that we find the need for God's healing. This woman who had given up said to me, almost like she had returned to her first love, "Today marks the beginning of coming back into the church."

What started as a simple request for mentoring turned into a living room full of open hearts that became a movement of women being real about their mess. Jesus met them there and so beautifully healed them and transformed their lives. That small group of girls invited a few friends who invited a few friends who invited thousands of friends to collide with Jesus, and it has been extraordinary to see God meet us in our brokenness and use us there too. If you had told me when I was hiding in the closet—so very hurt and a total mess—that God could use my pain to bring about beauty in other people's lives, I would have said that you were the crazy one. But that's what Jesus does. He leaves you more whole than broken, and then you leave others more whole than broken.

If I could, I would invite you into my living room and listen to your story, or I would open the door of that closet you're hiding in and sit with you there. But for now I want to invite you, in your story of beauty and brokenness, to walk alongside me in mine. I invite you to run into the One who brings wholeness to all this woundedness. Instead of running away from your pain, come with me, and we will run right into the One who can handle it and heal it. The One who changed me and still changes me can change you too. When He collides with us, we are never the same and neither are the people we run into.

So, I have this crazy hope . . . Imagine the possibility of you and me experiencing healing, even if little by little. Imagine no longer having to run and hide and pretend and deal with pain the way you have been taught. Imagine no longer trying to heal yourself in ways that cause more pain. Instead, picture running toward real healing. Imagine becoming more whole and imagine how that would change all our collisions. Rather than bringing pain to people who are already hurting, imagine us bringing healing instead. Instead of wounded collisions, imagine running toward healing ones. Imagine this being what we all need, what our world needs, to see all this brokenness sent packing.

Let's collide.

part 2

running into a healing God

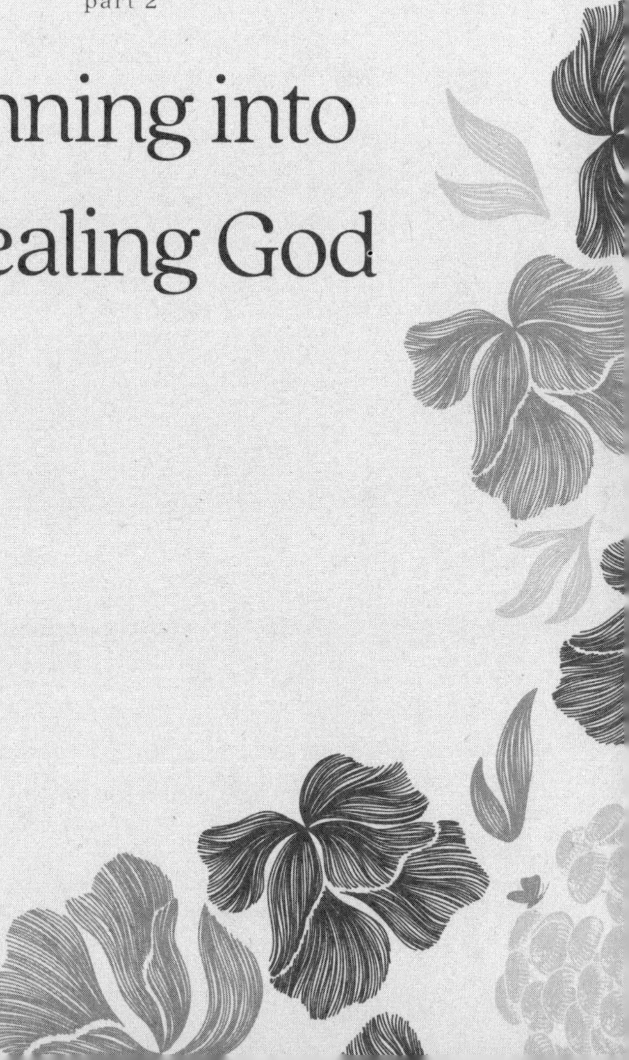

7

i'm not fines

In fifth grade, I got called into the principal's office. You know when you get called into the principal's office, it's never good. But this time I wasn't in trouble for ditching school to go to the candy store. This time I got called in to talk to a counselor.

They had received calls from people concerned about what was going on in my home, so the principal said I had to come in every Friday and I shouldn't tell home. I didn't tell home about the counselor, and I didn't tell the counselor about home. When I think back to being made to sit there every week, not feeling fine but pretending to be, I see a girl who knew exactly why she kept silent. I did all of us a favor and told a nice story that would be easier for everyone. It wasn't that I didn't know how to put words to what was going on. It wasn't that I thought I was fine. It's just that you and I can barely handle that we aren't fine, and we don't think others can handle it either.

Many of us aren't fine. We soak our sorrows in gin and juice, and we wish our days away with unconscious scrolling. We aren't speaking to our neighbors, and we are screaming at our kids. We keep calling ourselves the names *they* called us. We self-sabotage so other people can't hurt us. We are chronically insecure. We have broken hearts, ungrieved grief, and serious PTSD. And we're too afraid to go back to the place we experienced the trauma—it might kill us all over again. So, we just don't deal. We want to be like Kristen, and Kristen, she wants to be like Jenny, and Jenny wants to be like Megan, and none of us can ever rest and just be ourselves. We have skeletons in our closets, baggage we carry, and demons we fight. We have created rifts we can't seem to mend, and we have run from things that are now too far gone to fix. We have depression, stress, and fear—and meanwhile, we are all acting like we're fine.

The checker scans our organic carrots and our gallon bottle of vodka while asking, "How are you?" And we say, "Fine. How are you?"

Plagued by her own heartache, she bags our chicken and our cheese and answers robotically, "I'm good. Only six more hours . . ."

My husband, Rob, once went on a trip to India, and while serving at one of Mother Teresa's orphanages, he noticed a friendly boy walking around talking with the Americans. With a big smile this kid robotically said, "How. are. you. I. am. fine. How. are. you. I. am. fine." He looked like a two-year-old, but he was actually four. He was malnourished and anything but fine, yet he had been coached to say he was by an English-speaking group or individual.

We, too, have been taught to give canned answers rather than to share the truth. We live in a culture that values fake strength over being real. We pretend we're awesome rather than getting help when we're not. We avoid conflict even if it means faking relationships. We numb our not-fineness with Wordle, work, TikTok, retail therapy, porn, and rosé. We not only like fine, we prefer fine. We sell fine. Our profiles dish it up, and the more we look it, the more people follow us. We like fine so much we travel to other countries in Jesus' name and teach malnourished orphans to say they're fine, in our language, not theirs.

Sadly, even some of us Christians have modeled this wounded cultural value of "we're fine," "we're good," "we've got this," when we aren't, we're not, and we don't. The very people whose foundation is laid upon the belief that we are wounded, messy, fallen, sinful people in need of a God to rescue us are instead often walking around like we no longer need rescuing. We have all the answers, we are strong, we are right. We are the poster children of fineness. We once were lost, but now we're found. And we are going to tell everyone else how lost they are.

So, let's just level the ground right now. We *all* have struggles. Regardless of religion or lack thereof, age or race, hype or following, socioeconomic class or relationship status—we all have brokenness and baggage. Whether it's our neighbors, our coworkers, the Suzy Qs at church, the people we parent alongside, the chick whose house looks like Joanna Gaines's . . . let's not kid ourselves, they have struggles too. Some of us might be better at pulling ourselves up by our bootstraps. Some might be better at pretending. Some might be in a better season. But we all have "stuff" that makes us not fine.

You know what this "I'm fine" thing is, right?

Let me illustrate: I have a real bladder problem, so I find myself in bathrooms a lot. Maybe it's anxiety. Maybe it's a fear of peeing my pants on stage. Maybe it's drinking way too much coffee. I once walked into a public restroom, and there stood two women in their forties staring at me as if it was weird to be in the bathroom, so I asked if they were in line. They said, "Noooo," like it was a dumb question, so I squeezed past them only to realize they were cornering a teenage girl. I made my home in a stall while I heard this conversation play out . . .

The teenage girl's mom said all super judgy to her friend, "Do you knoooow what I called you in here to tell yoooou?"

Silence.

When the mom's friend realized what the mom was getting at, she said in that condemning voice we all can't stand, "How far aloooonng?"

The tension was thick as these two women competed in the shame-fest I apparently bought tickets for. Humiliated and sheepish, the teenage girl stuttered, "I . . . I . . . I'm . . . two months along."

More silence.

I was done peeing at this point and awkwardly trying not to interrupt this conversation that I think they forgot I was present for. The mom, with utter disdain and disgust over her daughter's pregnancy, said to her friend, "Your face tells me how you feel, and that's how I feeeel about it too." It was like their agreement about how repulsed they were ended the conversation, and then the three of them walked out and sat down, waiting to hear the preacher preach.

I pulled up my dreadful Spanx, flushed, washed, prayed—and then went and preached my heart out about a God who did the impossible through Mary, a pregnant teenager.

I bet this young girl's circumstance felt so overwhelming. I am sure she was scared, maybe full of regret, carrying a two-month-old burden. But neither woman asked how she was doing or expressed a willingness to walk alongside her. She told her truth, and she got slapped upside the head with, "You should be ashamed of yourself, you little . . ."

Look, I'm a mom. And I hope I never have to navigate this kind of situation with my daughter. God knows I wouldn't be like, "Oh I have always wanted to be a grandma while you were still in high school. Let's go buy some baby clothes." But God help me if I ever corner my kid and shame her. We don't have to abandon truth, but if we want people to invite us into where they really are, we better rethink our responses. Because I am pretty sure the next time that girl who got shame slapped is asked, "How are you?" she is sure to say—like the boy from India—"Fine. I am fine."

Maybe what happened in this bathroom is exactly why we all keep pretending we are fine. I want us to collide with a God who can handle our "I'm not fines," who will meet us right where we are, and who calls us to respond like He would when others aren't fine.

There's a story in the Bible where Jesus collided with a paralyzed man who, like us, could have easily said, "I'm fine."[1] But the most beautiful thing happened when he didn't. Jesus was back in His hometown, preaching to a packed house. The tickets were sold out. No one else could get into the living room. The place was drawing fans like Elvis had come back to life and was doing a house show.

The story goes, "Some men came, bringing to [Jesus] a paralyzed man, carried by four of them."[2] We don't know if these men were friends or strangers. But some kind of interaction had to have occurred for this paralyzed man to go from lying on a mat to being carried. The Bible doesn't say, "Some men came, dragging to Jesus a paralytic having a temper tantrum."

Most likely their encounter started off like most of ours do, with a "Hey, how are you?" I imagine this guy could have been thinking, *How am I? I'm paralyzed. Every time I get an inkling to do something, I'm at the whim of someone else.*

The man must have indicated he wanted to be carried. For a lot of us, letting people into our pain, our story, our needs, feels vulnerable and risky. Yet risking vulnerability was this man's first step toward the healing he longed for. The alternative was staying sick, alone, and stuck. This man knew he needed to get somewhere and couldn't get there on his own.

The Bible challenges our fear of getting hurt, our need to self-protect, and our tendency to run solo. It tells us to "carry each other's burdens, and in this way you will fulfill the law of Christ."[3] The law of Christ is not *going to church*. It's not *long prayers* and *virginity*. It's not *good works* and *voting the right party*. Nor is it smiling a lot, paying your taxes, and wearing turtlenecks up to your ears to cover your cleavage. The fulfillment of "the law"—or what Jesus holds as conduct of highest importance—is to carry for others what is oppressive, afflicting, worrisome, grievous, and too much to bear. And let's be honest, we don't want to be burdened by what burdens others.

We also don't want to burden others with what burdens us. We want to get better on our own. We want to wake up on a Wednesday and be whole. We want God to wave the magic wand so we can watch all the pain go away without bothering a soul. We definitely don't want to invite someone to carry what we carry and risk getting shame slapped. We'd rather stay alone in the struggle, and yet Jesus invites us to let people carry our burdens.

But guess what? People can't carry your burdens if they don't know what they are.

I am not sure why Jesus asks those of us who've been *hurt* by humans to *trust* humans when we're burdened. As crazy as it sounds, it's *people* He will use to help heal us. Our trust in others, our sense of safety, and our belief in the necessity of relationships all need to be made whole too. And I get it: This kind of trust takes the gutsiest guts you've got.

One of the most incredible things about the paralyzed man's collision with these four men is that they must have given him permission to be real about his need. There was no other way they could have carried him. We often posture a strength that can't handle weakness or inconvenience, a religious snobbery that judges, a purity incapable of touching anything dirty, a self-righteousness that puts sin on the defense, and a lack of safety that guarantees we will gossip about someone's burden like everything else. And when we posture these things, we will never be trusted with other people's burdens. But it seems these men postured the ability to handle pain just like their Lord did. So this man got real. And what was real was that he was *not fine* and he needed to be carried to the One who could handle his "I'm not fines."

When the men got to the packed house party and couldn't fit through the front door, they *unroofed the roof.* Most of us don't even climb the ladder, but they did whatever it took, at whatever cost, with whatever energy. It wasn't about them, and they all knew it. It was about a man who invited others into his story, and his story needed Someone Greater.

We don't carry each other aimlessly. We carry each other to the One who can handle what we can't. We unroof roofs to lower each other to collide with Jesus, who will, in the middle of a raging party, stop for one.

Imagine how exposed this man must have felt, in all his vulnerability and weakness, in all his incapability and need, as he was being lowered down to Jesus. The carriers had to have been second-guessing this move too. *What if Jesus doesn't help? What if people laugh? What if we drop him?* But there's just something about Jesus, something that makes us take big risks.

The Bible says, "Jesus saw their faith."[4] That's fascinating. Jesus saw the faith it took to be carried and the faith it took to carry. He saw the incredible strength and belief it took to say, "I can't do it on my own." Jesus honored the paralyzed man for getting real with himself, others, and God, which tells us Jesus will honor us for getting real too. Jesus also saw the incredible faith it took to carry this man. It takes faith to believe God can use you in your brokenness to help someone else in theirs. It takes faith to trust that the work is worth it. It takes faith to believe that Jesus can do something about what you can't.

Jesus then called the man who couldn't move "Son."[5] He first took care of what had been paralyzing this man's soul and forgave him. Jesus knew that this man had more going on than just physical and emotional pain. Whatever it was this man carried, one thing was for sure: Jesus wanted to heal it all.

And wouldn't you know it, there were some religious guys at the party talking trash about Jesus. He calls them out and then says to the paralytic, "I tell you, get up, take your mat and go home."[6] And this man walked out of there with a swagger.

It's mind-blowing what Jesus can do when we get real about our "I'm not fines."

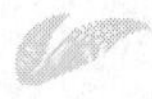

One afternoon my phone rang, and when I picked it up, I heard a woman's voice that I vaguely recognized. She began to explain an experience she had at one of our early Collide events. I hadn't planned on starting a *thing*, but apparently *God* started a thing. As I was being real about my pain, women started coming and being real about theirs. This woman on the phone said that for the first time in her sixty-five years, she was invited to be real about her story with other women.

So, at the event, she shared something she had never told anyone—not even her husband or her closest friends. She turned to a woman next to her . . . and told the hard, painful truth. She had gotten pregnant as a teenager, and her family sent her away to have her baby hush-hush. She was forced to give it up for adoption. When she returned home, she had been silenced, not allowed to share for fear of judgment and shame.

This woman had thought about her baby
every
single
day
for
fifty
years.

This woman had experienced a wounded collision with Christian parents who needed her to look perfect on the outside—even if it meant lying, pretending, and living in shame on the inside. She was like the sixty-five-year-old version of the teenager in the bathroom. This woman's entire life had been riddled with secrets, regret, and longing. She was not fine. But she experienced a new kind of collision, one where she was invited to be real, knowing that Jesus could handle her whole story. And this was why she called—to tell me that this was the beginning of healing for her. The moment she shared her story, she was changed.

Telling your story is where healing starts.

What if that pain you have felt for way too long could finally experience some relief? What if your first step toward wholeness is letting others in? What if the healing you long for is one "carry" away?

What if I had walked out of that closet and pretended I was fine? What if this mom who missed her baby every day for fifty years had kept silent the rest of her life? What if the teenage girl had said "I'm fine" instead of "I'm pregnant"? What if the paralytic had decided to pose as fine rather than inconvenience the bros? What if we *all* keep acting like we're fine when we aren't?

Then women who hide in closets, afraid of their alcoholic mothers, will pass their pain right on to their daughters. Then women who've missed their babies for decades will do it alone, and that's like giving your soul up for adoption. Then teenage girls who are far from fine will feel they can't tell us otherwise, and we won't get the privilege of walking alongside them. Then people who are stuck, unable to move, won't be picked up and taken where they need to go. Then we will keep missing out on what the power of a collision with Jesus can do when we carry each other to Him.

Fine keeps you on the mat. *I'm not fine*—getting real, being vulnerable, sharing your story as it really is, being brave enough to let people carry you—that will get you lowered down before the only One who can heal us all.

8

drunkards, gluttons, and swingers

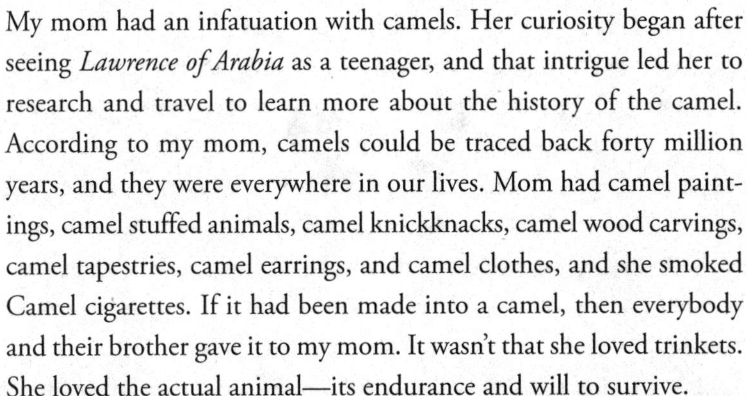

My mom had an infatuation with camels. Her curiosity began after seeing *Lawrence of Arabia* as a teenager, and that intrigue led her to research and travel to learn more about the history of the camel. According to my mom, camels could be traced back forty million years, and they were everywhere in our lives. Mom had camel paintings, camel stuffed animals, camel knickknacks, camel wood carvings, camel tapestries, camel earrings, and camel clothes, and she smoked Camel cigarettes. If it had been made into a camel, then everybody and their brother gave it to my mom. It wasn't that she loved trinkets. She loved the actual animal—its endurance and will to survive.

You know how some people sponsor children? Well, my mom sponsored a camel in California named Irvine. She got pictures and letters about her adopted animal and thought it a fantastic idea to have her artist friend BJ sketch it and then have it painted on the side of the café. This mural is now a tourist attraction. You will instantly recognize it if you've ever watched the popular '90s TV show *Northern Exposure*. Every episode begins with a shot of a moose walking down a street in Roslyn, Washington, pausing right in front of Mom's camel surrounded by palm trees, mountains, clouds, and the words "Roslyn Cafe An Oasis."

An oasis is a pleasant place that is surrounded by something unpleasant.

The old coal miners and I would eat breakfast at the café. They would cut my ham, and we would play tic-tac-toe on napkins. They would let me win. Every. Time. They were such sweet liars. At lunch, the guys from the lumberyard would come in and charm the waitresses. During summer, bikers would swarm the café. I had never seen so many tattoos in one place until I waited their tables.

Mr. and Mrs. Brand, my second-grade teacher and her husband, were regulars. There was also Tom, the waiter, who was as loving as he was crazy. He partied like it was 1999 in 1986, 1987, 1988 . . . any chance he could get, really. He had insane stories that entertained *and* scared me. There were the Seattleite yuppies who came over on the weekends to escape city life and made the café their first stop. There was Zandu, a local artist who creeped me out. Sporting a ponytail under her chin, she ate under her psychedelically simple swirl canvases that hung for sale on the walls. You know the kind. You look at them and think, "I could make that." This was my dining room growing up, and these were the people eating in it.

Looking back at this hodgepodge hippie hub of a meeting place, I wonder if this is the kind of spot where Jesus would have gone for a great mushroom burger and good company. Dining with all walks of life: strangers, liars, drunks, freak shows, and even kids—that's the kind of eating I imagine Jesus in the rhythm of. He is described in the Bible as "the Son of Man [who] came eating and drinking."[1] He even told us what kind of parties we should be hosting: "The next time you put on a dinner, don't just invite your friends and family and rich neighbors, the kind of people who will return the favor. Invite some people who never get invited out, the misfits from the wrong side of the tracks."[2]

You'll often see Jesus colliding with Judgy Judgertons who shame Him for the characters He's hanging with. One story in particular tells of Jesus colliding with a guy named Levi who was sitting in a tax collector's booth.[3] I don't know about you, but I picture Levi sitting in what looked like a lemonade stand. Maybe it was the first time they collided, but more than likely, Levi had at least heard about this Jesus guy. Jesus' reputation did always seem to precede Him.

Levi was a tax collector, and tax collectors' reputations preceded them too. Jesus colliding with Levi while he was on the job was like catching Levi right when he was stealing cookies from the cookie jar. Tax collectors used their power to bully, lie, and manipulate to amass wealth for themselves. They couldn't be witnesses in a court of law and were considered a disgrace to their family members. They were hated—so much so that they were not allowed in the synagogue to worship God and no one would dare eat with them.[4]

The voices of the surrounding social and religious culture likely affected how Levi viewed God and how Levi assumed God viewed him. So, it must have been quite the surprise when Jesus, who many called "Rabbi," invited this tax collector to follow Him. And as nuts as it was, Levi followed Jesus, leaving everything—stability, comfort, relationships, reputation, political alliance, and even the cookie jar.

Most of us have had really bad days at work, and we've thought about saying, "You can take this job and shove it." But Levi quitting on his boss? That was crazy talk. Levi worked for Herod Antipas, who was not a guy you wanted to mess with. Not only did Levi say sayonara to a man who beheaded guys like John the Baptist, he also left his bread and butter and maybe his Tesla, his time-share in Cabo, and his 401(k).

Jesus showed up to the party celebrating Levi leaving his old life to start a new one. When the religious teachers—the Pharisees—saw the bohos Jesus was laughing it up with, they kicked up a fuss. You can just feel the sneers and see the eye-rolling of the self-righteous orthodox in this room. Jesus at a hootenanny seemed asinine to those who were forbidden to hang out or do business with sinners.[5] These stuffy, pious snobs got all up in Jesus' grill. In this culture, eating with someone said, "We're friends," and devout people would never have said that to the likes of Levi.

The Pharisees were often labeled as "separatists" because they separated themselves from people who did not live as they did.[6] They believed segregation was the way to salvation. It was their attempt to avoid wounded collisions with broken humans who were messy and sinful. They ate with other people who lived as they lived, believed as they believed, worshiped as they worshiped, and valued what they valued. These religious people had a wounded view of God and a wounded view of people, which led to some serious spiritual eating disorders.

It strikes me that maybe we do too.

Many of us don't "eat" with people who are always down on their luck, people who are chronically depressed, people who interrupt like crazy, and people who burn us out. We like to be friends with people we think are charming, funny, intelligent, and beautiful . . . but not *too* intelligent or beautiful. We prefer people who cheer us on and make our golf game look good. Anyone who doesn't is invited last for bunco parties.

Many of us don't "eat" with people who could contaminate us. We think other people might "rub off" on our kids or "influence" our husbands. Their ignorance will make us look uneducated. Their rebellion will make us look less godly. So we wave, smile, and maybe say, "Hey, we should get together sometime" but then never do.

Many of us don't "eat" with people who invalidate us. We have zero tolerance for conversations that poke our belief bear. We invite people to dine with us who validate our theology, doctrine, and lifestyle. We invite them for Easter if they share the same sense of humor, the same voting record, and the same love of ham and Jesus. If we think people will invalidate our "God," our politics, or our comfortably held stereotypes, we just won't have them over for steak and potatoes.

We all seem to find ways to separate tribally. Our superclusters, our fences, our factions, and our fractures drive us farther and farther away from each other, toward those who are just like us. We put each other in boxes we never plan to open. Conservatives don't have liberals over for taco night. Liberals don't invite the conservatives over for crab feeds. Christians don't have BBQs with Muslims, and Muslims don't have burgers with Mormons, and Mormons don't have coffee with anyone.

We avoid the awkwardness of difference. The gathering of unlike people is becoming a rarity, and yet this is where you'd find Jesus colliding. Jesus' invite list brought together the diverse round the same table. If you want to hang with Jesus, He is hanging out at places like the Roslyn Café.

Jesus eats with the misfits, and He pulls out a chair for you too.

There was something about Jesus that was so beautiful, so magnetic, so poignant that people from all walks of life were drawn to Him. They journeyed far and long to get to Him, and they felt absolutely welcome. And you know what? Somewhere along the way, many of Jesus' followers lost sight of who He is. We lost sight of Jesus' mercy that handles messiness, His compassion that sits in people's pain, and His presence that though most holy, shows up in the unholiest of places to call outsiders "beloved."

Jesus calls us to invite into our lives not just our friends but the people we write off. They can't pay you back with social capital or spiritual ego boosts. But it's at this kind of party that Jesus shows up with His beauty, His magnetism, and His poignancy, RSVP'ing yes to the misfit table again and again.

If you're hungry for that kind of table, you're hungry for Jesus. Because that's where He's sitting. If you're feeling sneers from separatists, if you're failing to get the invite from religious folks, if you were hoping someone would stand up for you when you were being judged and they didn't, don't you ever forget about the God of the misfits.

If you find yourself only sitting at tables with people just like you, I'm going to turn the heat up at this party. You cannot call yourself a Christ follower and *not* gather round tables with people who don't look like you, act like you, believe like you, or vote like you. If you look at the life of Christ, you cannot escape that He did not escape humanity. Tax collectors and adulteresses, the pious and the irreligious, the zealous and the outcast all fell in love with Jesus. When? When He hung out with them.

God, in all His holiness, sits down with us, in all our unholiness. He sits across from our quirks, our stupid jokes, our halitosis, our ignorant opinions, and our stuffy theology. He keeps company with our impatience, our attempt to control the conversation, our dreadfully boring presence, and the spinach in our teeth.

The significance of Jesus eating with humanity is that the Sculptor of Mount Everest in all its splendor joins us for eggs and ham and calls little ol' us "chum." The God who paints a new canvas every sunset sets down His paintbrush, picks up His fork, gathers round the table with people as faded as we are, and calls us "dear." Jesus is not a "Wow, we should get together sometime soon" God. Jesus is a God who sits down with us, in all our humanness, and has wine and matzo balls, grapes and good cheese with crackers.

Now that is significant.

Jesus responded to the judgy people at this party in a pretty profound way: "It is not the healthy who need a doctor, but the sick."[7] Jesus knew that by sharing a meal with people who had begun to believe that God wanted nothing to do with them, He would show them otherwise. Jesus knew that when He reclined with those who never got an invite, He would heal their self-image that had been sickened by wounded collisions. But it wasn't just the "sinners" who were sick at this soiree. The Pharisees were feverish. They had a wounded view of God and neighbor. And Jesus wanted to heal it because it was hurting people He loved.

Jesus went on to say, "I have not come to call the righteous, but sinners."[8] I never heard about sin growing up. I hadn't heard that it deserved punishment or how to get rid of it. Though no one ever used this word or put a definition on it, I knew what sin was. You know sin because you live with humans, and even if you can't pinpoint it or call it something, you live in its air.

I remember a waitress named Miss You'llNeverKnowHerName who worked at my mom's café. She couldn't have kids with Mr. You'llNeverKnowHisName. Over time, she poured coffee for a regular at the café and realized that maybe he could help impregnate her. So this waitress and her old man agreed that on Tuesdays she would hook up with SpermDonor and try to make babies. So every week as a kid, I would smirk to myself, *Iiiit's Tuuuuesday!*

Miss You'llNeverKnowHerName ended up getting pregnant, falling in love with SpermDonor, and leaving Mr. You'llNeverKnowHisName. A few years down the road, she changed her mind and went back to him, tossing her kid to and fro between the two men. Even as a little girl who didn't know that most people's parents were married, I knew there was something whacked about swapping sex and confusing children as to who their father was.

My own father would roll into town every once in a blue moon and covertly slide an envelope stacked thick with hundies to my mom. It seemed like his way of thanking her for raising me. One time after he handed my mom a fat wad, he whisked me off to a Youngbloods concert. Afterward, he dropped me off at home and took off in his red Cadillac convertible. I watched him depart like I watched all his departures, never knowing exactly when I would see him again.

The town drunk, Lanky Louie, spent most of his time in my childhood mind at the local bars. Every time I saw him, he was drunk, and I wanted nothing to do with him. So you can imagine how grossed out I felt in junior high when I found this alky in my mom's bed one morning. Years later, Lanky Louie ended up passing out on the train tracks and died. Even as a kid, I had a deep sense that his wounds, his sin, his thirst stole his life out from under him. And no one needed to tell me that. I was sin's witness.

I had this friend whose stepdad would whip off his belt and use it to shame her right in front of me. He was a mean and awful man, and though no one said it, I knew he wasn't how a father should be. After the beatings, we would go out and play and forget it ever happened . . . until it was time for her to go back home. And then we both remembered.

I used to get a ride to school from another friend's house every morning. And every morning, her parents would get their giant bong out while we waited for our ride. They needed that hit to start their day. And even though addiction seemed normal, I had a deep sense it shouldn't be.

For me, sin had no definition. It had feelings, experiences, memories, and names.

I grew up with sinners. So when I got older, I began to see that I too had the capacity to "sin," to create my own mess, to hurt others, to need something to get through my day, to numb my pain by self-medicating, to sleep with people for love, to judge others, and on it goes. Once I heard about Jesus, I could barely believe my ears. Someone told me He loved me, and I thought if Jesus could love the likes of me and my people, I might just love Him right back.

And that's what got this sinner to love a Savior.

I often think back to my little town and the characters who shaped me, and I think these are the exact people Jesus would want in His living room. It was almost like Jesus showed up at that party to let all of humanity know how God truly feels about sinners.

I sin and you sin. We don't need religion to call our sin by name. We feel the pain of sin. We long for the presence that sin took away. We drink in the hopes that one more sip might remove the scars that belt left long ago. We regret getting angry, and then we get more angry that our rage is a result of our dad's rage and his dad's rage, and it's maddening that we can't make it stop. The people we so often label as "sinners"—they don't need you to convince them of sin. They live with sin's wounds.

Sinners need you to convince them of a Savior's love.

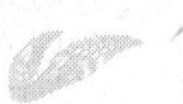

So friend, if you have been wounded by being told you're too wounded for Jesus, too much of a sinner for Jesus, too dirty, rotten, and no good for Jesus, then might I remind you what my soul needed for healing. We have a God who wants to sit across from us even if we pass out in our huevos rancheros, even if we cheat at tic-tac-toe, even if we are the judgiest Judgertons of them all. He is a God who wants to enter our lives—with our belt-swinging anger, Tuesday night swinger plans, and all. He is a God who invites the dads who have been gone far too long and the kids who have run away from home to come have supper with Him. Jesus chooses to experience the sneers of the religious, all to be with the town drunks and the bong-hitters. Contrary to all that you have been told, God wants to break bread with you, even if you're a misfit. Jesus came for sinners and said, "Let's have dinners."

9

wanting to be wanted

It was a common routine in my early years to put myself to bed because Mom had to close the café. The stools and chairs had to be put up so the floor could be mopped. The tips had to be counted. The grill had to be cleaned, the morning's breakfast prepped. The Rolling Stones had to be blasted. And the staff had to party when they got it all done. I would say good night to everybody, walk down the hall and up the long flight of stairs to our apartment, and tuck myself in by my night-light—the café's neon sign.

One night, I was startled out of a deep slumber in all the obnoxious ways you never want to be. In their drunken stupor, my mom and her boyfriend wanted dessert. The guy, in general, was weird. One Halloween he thought it would be creative to put a squash over his head as a costume. I mean, I would kind of get it if it had eye and mouth holes. But it didn't. His whole face was covered by a squash. My mom was dating Squash-Head Guy.

They came home after a night of partying, woke me up, and demanded I go downstairs to the café kitchen and make a hot fudge sundae. (The café did have the best hot fudge this side of heaven.) But I was tired. And I was five. So instead of being a good little waitress, I slept on the job.

Things got ugly. I refused to do what they demanded and packed some clothes into my little white plastic suitcase. This Squash-Head loser let me know that it was just fine for me to leave. My drunk mom didn't stop him. And she didn't stop me.

I drifted down Second Street in the middle of the night, toting my suitcase and a heavy sense that I had no idea where I was going.

No usual bustle of cars and bikes and stray dogs. No jaywalkers getting their mail at the post office. No shop owners doing business. No kids looking to play. All was still.

I scanned my little-kid mental file of people I could turn to for help. There was only one person on that list, and I was walking away from her.

The open road was lit by the moon. I looked up and let the snowflakes kiss my face. The sky in Roslyn might be the most beautiful vault of heaven you'll ever see. I mean, I know we share the same sky, you and I. But the Roslyn sky is full of stars, hemmed in by evergreens—almost like they embrace you, in moments when all you need is to be held.

Oscar Wilde wrote, "We are all in the gutter, but some of us are looking at the stars."[1] Sometimes, looking up is all we can do, when we're five and when we're forty-five.

Someone else said, "God writes the gospel not in the Bible alone, but on trees and flowers and clouds and stars." The only gospel, or good news, I had in that moment was in the constellations, the ridge that hemmed me in, and the moon that told me, despite how insignificant I felt in its light, I was not alone.

What I wanted was someone to swoop me up and hold me safe. Every step down that road found me wanting to be wanted. And that led to me walking down so many other painful roads, for years, hoping someone would care. You could take a snapshot of my life at any number of mileposts, and you'd see me doing whatever it took in the hopes that someone would come for me.

I think back to my move-in weekend as a college freshman. I got wasted the first night, and I ended up back in my dorm room doing things I now regret because a girl who wanted to be loved ran into a boy who wanted to be pleasured. This wanting-to-be-wanted feeling has found many of us walking down roads that end up making us feel less wanted.

This is where the woman in John 8 was.[2] Her deep desire to be wanted led her down a road that made her feel less wanted than ever. And it was right there, at her seemingly least desirable, that she and Jesus collided.

Jesus was teaching in the Temple at the crack of dawn. I am a firm believer that nothing good happens before 9 a.m. But here these people were, gathering to hear Jesus when it's "too a.m." for me. And wouldn't you know it, some "spiritual leaders" dragged a woman in like trash and placed her right before Jesus. Here He was, halfway through His sermon, when they made a spectacle of her, shaming her with "This girl is a no-good, dirty tramp! She was caught in the act of adultery!"

Awkward. No formal introduction. Just, "Jesus . . . Tramp. Tramp . . . Jesus."

These religious guys who thought they had this woman all figured out thought they had God all figured out too. They claimed God commanded them to pummel her to death with stones. They met this woman on mile nine, and they summed up her entire worth based on one stretch of highway named "I Blew It."

We all do this. We collide with people at whatever milepost they happen to be at, and we make assumptions without considering all the roads that led them there. My husband and I met with our daughter's potential teacher. We sat down on kiddie chairs across a kiddie table from Mrs. NotWhoIExpected. The whole experience was supposed to give us the warm fuzzies about leaving our baby at school for the first time. I'll be honest, I definitely had a stereotype of what my kid's teacher would be like: the apple-pin-and-cardigan-wearing, calm-voice chick who sleeps at her desk and for a hobby spends time at the library.

And she was warm, and she was friendly. But right after she asked if our kid was allergic to anything, my husband said, "You look really familiar." When my husband says things like this, I get nervous and for good reason: He also used to be a lil' wild. The teacher said, "You look really familiar too." They figured out that they had gone to the same college at the same time. Rob squinted his eyes to guess what she looked like fifteen years prior. She did the same. I uncomfortably giggled and said, "Oh you probably don't recognize my husband. He was really crazy in college." They were still trying to make the connection, so I reminded us why we were all there, "Oh honey, I am sure she has other questions to ask us about our kid."

As soon as we left this ultra-awkward meeting, Rob said, "I know why she looks familiar!" And then he told me stories of his crazy past colliding with her crazy past, and I'll tell you this: They aren't the kinds of things you'd picture your kid's teacher doing. I was like, "Really? This is who will be reading *Goodnight Moon*, doing noodle art, and teaching the days of the week to my kid? Awesome."

We so easily pass judgment. We so easily label others and pick up stones. We have no clue what led them to the places we condemn. We don't acknowledge that where each person is today has a great deal to do with where they've been and what they've experienced.

Those men in John 8 were accusing the woman of *adultery*. The Greek phrase translated "caught in the act of adultery" originally meant "caught in the act of *theft*."[3] All the roads she had walked had led her to steal what wasn't hers in the hopes that she would be wanted.

This woman had every reason to assume Jesus would be exactly like the religious people condemning her. Because isn't that what we do? We make assumptions about God based on what we've experienced with His people. We assume God is as critical as the parent we could never please. We assume He is here to break up the party. We suppose God is just like "them," and "they" are the worst. We think He is as tired of us as we are of ourselves. We have all sorts of assumptions about God, and a lot of them have been informed by our wounded collisions.

This woman could only assume, by these angry men's certainty, that Jesus was also a torturer. And while they held so tightly to their stones, just waiting to pummel her along with everything they despised, hated, and disrespected, they too had assumptions. They clearly believed God only extends grace to people who don't mess up. Imagine that . . . grace extended only to those who never make mistakes. How is that grace again?

There stood Jesus, supposedly God in the flesh. If the people who represented God thought she deserved punishment, how much more would Jesus think so? Would He be like all the other men this woman had collided with? If men used her for their own pleasure, maybe Jesus would use her as an example? If townspeople judged her, maybe Jesus would too?

She didn't challenge the charge and neither did Jesus. This wasn't a case of "You've got the wrong girl." Jesus knew they were using her as a tool like every other man had, but this time it was to trap *Him*. It was a trap pitting mercy against justice, set in the sexual arena, and Jesus was supposed to take a side.

Where would Jesus place Himself? If He truly was a friend of sinners, wouldn't He side with mercy? But if He sided with mercy, wouldn't He be saying that adultery was OK? In that case, Jesus Himself would be condemned for contradicting the law. Jesus had already spoken publicly about this subject, and He actually raised the bar on what constitutes adultery, claiming, "Anyone who looks at a woman lustfully has already committed adultery with her in his heart."[4] So would Jesus side with justice? If He did, then what about Him being a friend of sinners?

This was the trap of all traps. One person would ultimately be condemned, and that One was Him.

Jesus could have said, "I am not going to fall for this. I'm outta here!" He could have given the woman a lecture on adultery, quoting Scripture and telling her how wrong she was. He could have left her to face the consequences by herself. But He didn't. Double underline this: Jesus didn't walk away from the trap because He would not walk away from the woman.

These legalistic men demanded, "What do You say, Jesus?"

Notice Jesus didn't feel the need to say anything right away. We live in a world where we feel like we have to respond to all the haters, but Jesus didn't feel the need to do that. Jesus bent down and wrote on the ground. And I wonder if in that moment Jesus saw all the roads this woman had traveled since she was a little girl. I wonder if Jesus knew what had led her from one road, to the next, to the next. I wonder if He knew why she so desperately wanted to be wanted.

All I know is that Jesus sees differently than we see.

Jesus knows the origin of our wounds, the collisions we've experienced, the lies we've picked up, the ways we've numbed our pain. He knows every last mile we've journeyed. And because He can see what we can't, His view has an expansive grace that understands how mile nine led to mile nineteen. He gets why No One Wants You Street led to Dumb Dorm-Room Boy Avenue. He knows how walking down a road alone at five years old will find you walking down all sorts of paths waiting for someone to come get you. Jesus sees where you are and how you got here, and He understands. He makes room for us to have hope in who we can become despite who and where we've been.

To the dismay of these self-righteous men, Jesus didn't take their side and grab the biggest stone. No, He invited these men to think about their own travels: "If any of you have never sinned, then go ahead and throw the first stone!"

We've all done things we're ashamed of. I can imagine each of these men realizing the weight of their own culpability.

The day after Rob and I got all judgy and self-righteous about our kid's potential teacher, our kids had soccer games, and afterward we went out for donuts. A family walked in, and boy did the man look familiar. I squinted my eyes and pictured what he might have looked like years prior. He did the same. Oh man—it was the guy from my first weekend in college. I immediately thought about the teacher I had judged. *Maybe I shouldn't wear cardigans either.*

Jesus stooped down again and began writing. People endlessly speculate about what He scribbled. The prophet Jeremiah says, "Those who turn away from you will be written in the dust because they have forsaken the Lord, the spring of living water."[5] So whose names were being written in the dust? These men held so tightly to their opinions that their opinions became weapons. They had forsaken God, and there was no greater evidence than how they treated this fellow human. I have a feeling it *was* these men's names that Jesus etched into the ground.

And wouldn't you know it, the would-be stone-throwers left one by one, each recalling a road they wished they had never walked down. Anytime we think we're better than someone else, Jesus helps us see that all our names are penned in the sand. All of us have forsaken God, fallen short of His glory, turned to the wrong things for love, and walked down roads that hurt us and others.

This woman had to be wondering if her punishment was still to come. Perhaps the worst punishment of all is to look Love right in the eyes and realize He'd been there all along. And not only had you completely missed Him, but your efforts to secure love elsewhere had hurt you and hurt Him.

Jesus asked, "Where are they? Has no one condemned you?" The woman looked around, and all those haters who thought she deserved death were gone. You can almost hear that she felt safer: "No one, sir." Jesus, our safest place, assured her in the same way I believe He assures you and me: "Neither do I condemn you."[6]

After this reassurance, Jesus said, "Go, and sin no more."[7] I had always read these words like He was yelling at me with a disapproving megaphone: "GO, AND SIN NOOOO MORE!" But I've had a change of mind. One commentator said Jesus' words were a charge for her to go and live differently.[8] William Barclay, a Scottish theologian, said, "In Jesus there is the gospel of the second chance. He was always intensely interested, not only in what a person had been, but also in what a person could be. He did not say that what they had done did not matter; broken laws and broken hearts always matter; but he was sure that everyone has a future as well as a past."[9] Jesus doesn't want any of us walking roads wanting to be wanted, only to end up feeling less so. Jesus believed about her what He believes about you. You are worthy of more—more than you have been made to believe, more than the standards you settled for, more than the miles you see in your rearview mirror.

And you know Jesus didn't just *say* you are worthy of more. Jesus *showed* you that you are.

You better believe Jesus chased this woman down every road she ever walked that led to this one. He collided with her in the moment when she felt the least lovable, least wanted, and least chosen. He knew that by standing with this woman, He would ultimately be condemned so she would be set free. But He showed up anyway. Jesus stood with her in her shame despite the pain it would cause Him. Jesus knew those haters would set out to kill Him since He wouldn't let them kill her. But He wanted to show her, with His life now and His death later, that she was worthy of it all.

Before she changed a thing, before she even confessed to walking down some sketchy roads, before she went and tried to sin no more, Jesus made sure she knew:

"You are already loved.

You are already chosen.

You are already worthy."

Once a girl knows that she is loved, chosen, and worthy, she knows she's wanted. She doesn't have to buy love at a discounted rate. She doesn't have to steal love from someone else. She doesn't have to walk down alleys, longing for someone to choose her. She doesn't have to drink to numb the pain of all the unwanted things she's done to feel wanted.

No, once she collides with Jesus and sees that He wants her more than His own life, she walks differently, sees differently, feels differently, lives differently. She no longer walks with a suitcase in hand, wondering where she is going. She walks knowing who her Father is, where her home is. She knows who she is and whose she is, so she can now roam those same streets telling other girls just like her, "You, girl, you are already wanted."

10

absence makes the heart

I have an old Polaroid of little kid me holding a picture of my dad. It's that classic retro-looking snapshot from my "Mom, why did you let me wear those clothes?" era. The photo I'm holding is worn from use and fairly big, probably eight by ten. Apparently I carried it everywhere, right alongside Cookie Monster and my blankie. I had heard that I had a dad and would meet him one day. This was him—he looked black-and-white, with stringy hair and a scraggly beard. Until he came for me, I clung to an image of him.

When I was maybe four, Mom drove me to visit this dad of mine. On that drive, the terrain began to change. The road became dusty. Barren, faded, lifeless. Even now, when I try to remember this meetup, I don't see his face.

I see lines.

Boundaries.

Fences. Lots of fences.

Instead of being scooped up, warm and close, I sat across a table from this strange man while he talked to my mother. Tough-guy rule keepers watched over us. Suddenly something struck my arm. I started screaming and swatting, flailing my arms about, creating a commotion. On the drive home, I could have closed my eyes and tried to remember my dad, but the only recollection I could muster was the real sting—of that bee.

A handful of years later, Mom took me to the Greyhound station that tripled as a motel and antique store. So if you ever needed a grandfather clock, a tacky place to sleep, and a slow ride to pretty much anywhere, this was your spot. Mom plopped eight-year-old me on the bus, said, "It's time to go visit your dad," and waved goodbye. I traveled a few hours and got off at the downtown Seattle station. For a small-town girl, the city was big-time. I stepped into a sea of travelers, looking for him. He greeted me, as he always would, with cheer, humor, and a groovy little arm dance (the kind daughters tell their dads not to do but secretly sort of love). And he looked like me, or I should say, I looked like him.

Our visits were odd. We were supposed to have a bond, and we both knew we didn't. Blood doesn't bond you. Neither does the same last name. I had my mom's last name anyway. My dad and I didn't have the father-daughter connection, and we were helplessly unsure how to get it.

One time, I had just arrived at my dad's house. His place was dingy and dark and smelled like mold. My white pants discovered a serious flea infestation, but more foreign for me was the poster of some steamy swimsuit model above the toilet. Mom would never have hung such a tasteless spectacle. While I was unpacking in my room, he got a phone call. He sounded alarmed. Something about "a murder . . . a limo . . . money . . . being 'next.'" I tried to keep my cool and pretend I hadn't heard and wasn't scared. I was good at that by then. Somebody should have given me a freaking Golden Globe.

My dad hurried into my room and said, "Pack up your things. You're getting back on the bus." No explanation, no fear relieved, just a direct order to skedaddle. He sent me back home to be a small-town girl, but this time, I wondered, *Would I ever see my big-city dad again?*

Months later, Mom said I was going back to Dad's for the weekend. I got out my white suitcase that was still sporting the last bag tag, the ink of my name beginning to wear off. I didn't want to go. Mom made me go anyway.

Our occasional visits were awkward for both of us. He had no idea how to be a dad, and I had no idea how to be a daughter. We were teaching each other, and our lessons were difficult. I was frightened of my dad, but I desired to be close. Maybe my dad felt the same. We did an awkward fright-desire dance on Fridays and ended up giving high fives and hugging on Sundays.

I wanted my dad to reeeealllly like me and even love me. And there were things about him that I liked too. He told fabulous stories and silly jokes, and I found him rather clever, hilarious, and highly interesting. My dad was more generous than anyone I have ever met. He helped those on their last dime—people everyone else would give up on. I grew up seeing this kind of grace in him and wondered if it was because he had needed it a few times himself. He always faced his circumstances with a "Life is good," posturing a positivity that would change the world if we were all to adopt it.

He and I would walk Green Lake, bike Lake Washington, and play cards. He mandated we watch *It's a Wonderful Life*. He also forced me to go see *E.T.* I thanked him afterward. It was a cold thanks that made sure he understood, "I'm glad we went to that movie, but don't you start thinking you know how to do this dad thing." He would hand me four to five hundred-dollar bills and drop me off at the mall, saying, "Have fun, Dot." (*Dot* was short for *daughter.*) This hippie kid discovered Nordstrom and fashion and the power of the Benjamin. Thank God. Otherwise, I'd still have unbrushed hair and be rocking hand-me-down flower child dresses over jeans, scuffing Moon Boots.

People flocked to my dad to hear him philosophize and to laugh at his humor. We were treated like celebrities when we visited his entrepreneurial endeavors. We went to meetups with bizarre characters. Record label execs, construction crewmen, twitchy cokeheads, porn stars, lawyers, restaurateurs, and strange girlfriends. Most, the kind you don't want to be around. One minute we were hanging out in a dive before hours, with me feeling like maybe we shouldn't be there, and the next we were at some bougie restaurant. He would say, "Bring me your best of everything." That's when I discovered calamari, Shirley Temples, three-hundred-dollar bottles of wine, cashmere, silk, Cadillacs, and schmoozy men. The people we sat across from would recollect stories, and Dad would look at me and back at his guest. Then in his cool way, Dad would remind them, "A kid is present, man." I got to buy fancy outfits for such occasions, and he would drive me in his beater truck to posh places and order exorbitant amounts of food and drinks and use really big words and ask, "Do you know what that means?"

"Have you seen pachyderms?"

"What's a pack E derm, Dad?"

"Elephants, girl. Elephants."

And then, as though the big words didn't make me feel dumb enough, he'd throw out a small one he was sure I didn't know.

"Boon. Know what a boon is?"

"Noooo, Dad," I'd say, rolling my eyes like they might never roll back.

"A boon is a gift. From the powers that be, kid."

"Do you know what braggadocio means, Dot?"

"No, Dad."

"It means boastful, arrogant."

"Funny. Aren't you being braggadocio right now, Dad?"

I never knew what those big, or small, words meant.

What I *did* know was that I wanted this dad to love me, to want me, to stay with me. I wanted it one minute, and the next I hated his guts and gave him a "Whoooo are yoooou, and wheeeere have you been all my life? You call yourself a daaaad?" attitude. After an interesting weekend, he would drop me off at the station to travel back to the way of life and the woman he once so quickly left.

I came home to Roslyn with new stories and a haul of new finds: a boom box, A. Smile jeans, a turquoise sweater dress, a turquoise spiked belt, and of course some rhinestone-adorned pink cowgirl boots. I was ready to be the coolest kid in school. Mom greeted me when I got off the bus. Clearly she had spent all day at the Pastime tavern, because she could barely walk, but there she was, my driver. The ladies at the front desk of the station were whispering. I could hear them questioning my ride. I questioned it too. Their concern, donned with a lack of action, felt like my old clothes, well-worn.

Every time I got in a car like that, I hated the life I couldn't do anything to change. If only it were as easy as getting some new threads.

Visits to my dad brought escape as much as they did pain. Each trip was a reminder that he knew little about me. I could see he was trying. Trying doesn't make up for what's been lost, but it's all you can do once you realize you didn't try hard enough.

This dad, I think he cared. I think he wished things had been different. But I needed more than that. The gifts, the money, the concerts, the trips, the cars, the jokes, the advice, the dictionary full of big words—sure, I liked all of it. Well, maybe not the dictionary. But what I really needed I couldn't have even told you at the time. All I knew was that I didn't have what it was.

We didn't have what it was.

I have spent years trying to put words to how I have been shaped by daily life without a dad, trying to understand the power of this absence. Maybe you have come up speechless about an abyss in your life too. The only way to articulate what my dad and I missed out on is that it looks like chapters and chapters and chapters we cannot get back, and their pages are blank . . .

Blank pages because there were few words.

Because there were minimal paragraphs.

Because there were hardly any chapters.

Because the story that could have been, that was supposed to be, was not.

Perhaps the power of absence can only be understood by the power of presence.

I have had front-row seats to watch my husband with our daughter. From her first bath to her first tears, he was there. He tucked her in every night. He bandaged her skinned knees. He went to every school musical and every stinkin' gymnastics meet. He holds her when she cries and makes her laugh on the good days and the bad. He gives her inspirational speeches before she has to do something brave. He tells her she is beautiful, and she believes him. She runs to him and envelops him with her whole self, and she says with all her heart, "I love you, Daddy," and he says back, "I love you, honey."

This is something I have never known. But I was made for it. I was intended to experience the kind of love that can be trusted to stay. And so were you.

As I try to put words to this gulf, I feel an unsatisfied sadness, a cutting regret, that I can't make disappear. We can never get the days back, the pages back, the chapters to do over. They are gone—in the archives of history, blank as blank can be. So I sit in the ache of absence, and it never seems to go away. It eats at me. I could cry at the drop of a hat for what could have been but never was. You might know this deep sadness too.

Those of us who have experienced the blank pages left by absence, death, separation, estrangement, infertility, debilitation, or crushed dreams share this ache.

Many try to say what absence makes the heart do.

Absence makes the heart wander.

Absence makes the heart grow fonder.

I say . . . absence makes the heart long prodigiously.

Do you know what *that* means?

Prodigious means remarkably vast in size, extent, power.[1]

You and I, we have a remarkably enormous longing that threatens to overpower us. We might not even know that we live out of it, trying to satiate the haunting emptiness.

Earlier, we met a woman who was deeply wounded by the blank pages that her circumstance penned.[2] In Mark 5, she had one of the most beautiful, life-changing collisions with Jesus that I have ever seen. A religious leader named Jairus fell at Jesus' feet, pleading that He heal his dying daughter. The Bible says, "So Jesus went with him."[3] I love that. I love that Jesus wasn't like, "Let me look at my calendar. Oh bummer. I have a one o'clock."

And right then, this woman who'd been bleeding for twelve years interrupted them. She had spent everything she had to get better but instead had grown worse. It's likely she was also socially outcast, emotionally downtrodden, and soul weary. She had every reason to believe God wouldn't show up for her. Her miracles had not come nor had her prayers been answered. She had probably told herself what I told myself every day in my blankie-draggin', Cookie Monster–totin', where's-my-dad era: *He probably won't come.*

That way, we don't get too disappointed.

We are hope temperers. This is how we self-protect. We've *had* to. Our hope has been let down for so many chapters that we brace for disappointment again in this one.

You know the feeling. I mean, how many times can you keep trying for the baby? And how many times can you show up as the third wheel, waiting to be someone's first choice? And how many times can you hope they come back, even though they never do?

For some reason this woman did what we least expect. She fought the crowd to get what she wanted. She came up behind Jesus and reached for healing. When's the last time you fought to reach the healing you hoped for? The Bible says her bleeding stopped immediately, and she was freed from her suffering. Jesus realized power had gone out from Him, so He turned around and asked, "Who touched my clothes?"[4] Why did Jesus care? He had places to go and a kid to heal and plenty of power where that came from.

I think Jesus wanted this woman to know that He saw her and always had. He had seen all the pages of her story. And He sees all the pages of ours. We have a God who is so personal. Scriptures say He knows our name. He knows the number of hairs on our head. He keeps track of our sorrows, collecting our tears in a bottle, recording each one in His journal. God knew the day you would be born, and He knows the day you will move to your forever home.[5] God knows your maiden name, your married name, and the names you call yourself. He knows the untapped gifts you're afraid to use. He knows the way you snort when you laugh and why you burst out crying in your car all alone. He knows you're allergic to pineapple, and that's why He made strawberries. God doesn't need a Find Your Friends app to locate you. He knows where you are, and He knows how you're doing, even when *you* don't know how you're doing.

Jesus stopped for this woman and gave her His unwavering presence. She fell at His feet and bravely told Him what Scripture calls her "whole truth."[6] And then we witness one of the most healing moments one can ever experience.

Jesus called her "Daughter."[7]

There is not a more personal name a father can use than one that says, "You are mine. And I am yours." The psalmist says God "determines the number of the stars and calls them each by name."[8] Our Father might call the stars by name, but He calls you:

"Daughter."

"Son."

"Kid."

I walked into church one Sunday, with my husband and kids in tow, and was taken aback. My good buddy Ron was doing his thang and started strumming to a song. The community of voices began to sing . . .

You tell me that You're pleased
And that I'm never alone

You're a good, good Father
It's who You are . . .
And I am loved by You
It's who I am[9]

The more they sang it, the more I wept. I looked like a Kardashian caught in a rainstorm, my makeup having a meltdown.

I'm still her. Forty-something and I'm still the girl carting around this hope that maybe, just maybe, I will be worthy of showing up for. And maybe you are carting this hope around too. Right there in like row twelve I said to God, *I just don't know how to do this. I don't know how to be a daughter.* This song identifies God as our Father, and as I sang it, I wanted it to identify me. I fell apart trying to sing. Rob reached his arm around me and pulled me tight. I dug down deep, and in what can be a vulnerable move for all of us, I reached for Him like I saw the hemorrhaging woman do. *God, teach me how to be a daughter. Help every cell of my body to believe I am loved by You . . . That it's who I am. Because it's who You are.*

Absence makes the heart go prowling round, doin' everything it can to fill itself. But a father's presence, *the* Father's presence, fills you so full that you need not long prodigiously because you know who you are. You're His kid. So if you're like me and you don't know how to do this dad thing, start by telling Him. Do the soul work of allowing your entire being to be loved by your Dad—your heavenly, perfect, present, good, loving Father.

I don't know what gaping hole absence has left in your life. I don't know what blank pages you wish were filled. But I do know that you and I have a Father who lets us interrupt Him at any hour. We can pull on the hem of His robe and tell Him our whole story. Whether it's the three thousandth time or the very first, He invites us closer, and the first thing He whispers is:

"You are mine."

11

rescue

In 1985 I was eleven. I was in my prime. I won a writing contest at school that sent me to the Young Authors Conference. I had written a book called *Willow's Whispers*, whose title I turned into an acrostic with stickers, on the cover that I made out of tinfoil. Stories of unicorns, of course, and frogs rescuing humans from a plane crash, and a mouse in my house eating my blouse all found me in an imaginary world that I created. I won the school spelling bee and then went to the state bee, earning a brand-spankin'-new dictionary for second place.

My dad would have been proud.

My friend Ronnie and I shot hoops for hours and then popped into the café or her house for a snack. Sometimes we hung out with her mom in her smoking room, where the couches were covered in plastic. I wondered what kind of special occasion allowed those covers to be lifted. And if there was going to be such an occasion, I wanted an invite. Her mom was the lunch lady at school. And it's always a good idea to be friends with the lunch lady.

Ronnie and I had vastly different experiences and yet shared a friendship that made room for difference. She had a white mom and a Black dad and five brothers. Every visit to her house was accompanied by a story, a lesson, or a sermon—and I mean that in a good way. I always felt like I walked out their door taught, pushed, and inspired.

It seemed to me that Ronnie was born with fight. I always wished I had what she had: this uncanny ability to handle whatever came her way, with a might that promised, "You cannot break me." I sometimes wondered if Ronnie had permission to be anything other than strong. This was the way to survive. For different reasons, I knew this too, but I felt much more breakable than she looked.

Ronnie's dad, Willie, was the local gravedigger and the school janitor. He had also served as the first Black mayor in Washington state. Ronnie's family was the reason for my first church experience. I was so excited about Sunday school that I skipped all the way home and knocked on the door to share my enthusiasm. Mom opened the door, and I belted out, "The B-I-B-L-E! Yes, that's the book for me! I stand alone on the Word of God, the B-I—"

Mom slammed the door.

On faith.

Willie was one of the most encouraging characters from my childhood. He would talk of God with reverence, as though God was real, without question. He always lectured us about doing the right thing, working hard, showing respect, honoring family. And he always sneaked in a "You gonna marry one of my sons someday?" This is how I knew he liked me. I knew he had my back if I ever needed it. But I also knew I would never trouble him. And I never did.

Willie always called me "Willa." He would say, "Willa, you're so pretty, but you gotta do something about that hair."

He was right. I've always wanted *your* hair.

Willie would sit in the dark and watch basketball with the temp cranked up in the basement. I always wondered why he liked to sit in a pitch-black sauna. I could only handle it for a few minutes, but I knew Willie had handled heat I'd never have to. He delivered powerful mini sermons the second we popped in, each one cranking up the heat on my life.

"Always do the right thing, always."

"Tell the truth. Don't you ever lie."

"You have one life. Whatcha gonna do with that one life, Willa?"

Never once did I dismiss his advice. I'd stand there with my heart saluting Willie. I knew this man not only practiced what he preached, he preached what he believed we had *in us* to practice.

Willie cleaned the school on weekends, and Ronnie and I would get the entire gym to ourselves. We'd play basketball, dreaming we'd take state champs in high school like the older girls we looked up to. We played around-the-world, and when we traveled its circumference a hundred times, we moved to bump, and when we got tired of bump, we played pickup games with the boys.

I pretty much peaked in middle school, people.

I wore black lace half gloves and made up dances to Madonna's songs. I learned how to breakdance. I loved shooting three-pointers as much as I liked boys. I looked in the mirror and liked what I saw, which might have been the last era this was true. I dressed up my cats, Bennie and Jet—named after the Elton John song—and posed them in a wheelbarrow with flowers like cat models. I took pictures of them, and that seemed normal. If it's not, I don't want to know about it. By the time I was thirteen, I wrote in my diary daily and named it after the boy I thought I loved. I played Bon Jovi's song "Never Say Goodbye" every night while thinking of him.

Play. Stop. Rewind. Nope, rewind a little more. Stop. Play. Stop. Rewind.

By fifteen, I found myself over at Aunt Jill's more. I guess I was growing more scared and more brave. I ended up kind of moving in the summer of freshman year. I slept in my cousin's room next to her bed. We didn't talk about why I was there. Andrea and I shared a love and a pact to protect one another that we never said with words, just actions. And we still do. Mom didn't ask me why I was camping out at Jill's. It worked for me, and I think it worked for her too.

I was visiting a family friend in Seattle for a weekend, and while I was there, my dad made me meet him. He took me for a walk and told me Mom insisted I move in with him. I was stunned. *My mom is getting riiiid of me?* I started to spiral. *Why didn't she talk to me first? I am the problem? Of course I am. Does anyyyyone care how I feel?* This news pulled the rug out from under all I knew. I knew Mom was a mess and I was struggling, but I never in a million years thought she would send me away.

My mom and I were never on the same page about why she wanted to do this. It was always my fault, not hers. I was a bratty teenager sneaking makeup in middle school and shaving my legs in the dark. I killed her parties, screaming at people, telling them to turn their music down, to get out, to *get a life!* When yet another drunk man became a regular in our house, I let him know what a loser he was. Exasperated by our patterns, I started putting voice to my insides. A furious fight was rising in me to change something, anything.

So yeah, I mean, I guess it was my fault. Because it's always my fault. I should have put up with all of it, covering addiction's lies. I should have been OK with hairy legs in high school and a drunk mom at basketball games. I should have accepted the gross men in her bed, and I should have been OK being alone night after night. I should have been OK with her wanting to party more than parent. So yeah, maybe she got rid of me because I was an ungrateful, judgy brat. Or maybe she was doing whatever she could to save us, and us being apart from each other seemed like salvaging any *us* we had left.

On that walk, I finally let my dad have a piece of my mind. My hatred of him and my blame, not for what he did but what he didn't do, came gushing out with an ugly vengeance: "I willll nevvvver live with *you*."

Now we both hurt, and it felt better that my hurt was no longer alone.

We often seek a companion for our pain without even realizing it. Maybe if my dad could feel how much it hurt to have someone you want to love you not choose you, he would feel how deep that cuts. Feeling like you're not worthy of being chosen, not worthy of presence, not worthy of keeping—that is a devastating feeling that never quite goes away. Maybe rejecting my dad was my revenge, or my comfort, or both. All I know is none of us like our pain to sit alone.

Dad and I both knew I shouldn't live with him. We both knew his life wasn't fit for a kid. And we both knew he wasn't gonna get his act together to make it suitable. So a distant aunt and uncle took me in. I moved out of my house before I got a driver's permit, before I made varsity, before we got to go to state, before the boy I wrote to every night confessed his undying love for me . . . before I wanted to.

It seemed like my best option. I would save myself before I was pawned off to who knows who. I would make my own choice. I remembered someone telling me when I was little that an alcoholic has to hit rock bottom in order to want to change. I think I believed I could bottom my mom out by leaving her. Maybe somehow losing me would rescue her. And if I could rescue her, maybe I could rescue me.

I left Roslyn almost like a protest, like I had learned from Martin Luther King Jr. and Jesse Jackson and the tree-hugger friends of my mom. Like, I will make a temporary stand, and then she will make a permanent change. I will sacrifice for the both of us, and she will realize our need for help. I wasn't being heroic. I was desperate.

So I said goodbye. I said goodbye to the café, the regulars, the cooks, and the mushroom burgers. To my favorite waitress, the miners, my cats, and my living room. To nicknames, team positions, and first chair in band. I said goodbye to Willie and to my friends Burt the Squirt and Heather and Ronnie. To Aunt Jill and my cousin Andrea, the nasturtiums and the big apple tree. To Friday night popcorn with brewer's yeast at the theater and to Saturday night high school cheers, chants, and hopes for more. I said goodbye to the tansies and the river, the stars in my sky, the trees on my ridge, and the cross on the hill. I said goodbye to my mom and the smell of her Oil of Olay, her cuddles and the I-L-O-V-E-Y-O-U's, our hugs, our talks, our *we*.

I said goodbye to all I loved without actually *saying* it. This goodbye crushed me, still crushes me. The mandatory farewells, the dismissal, the feeling of being tossed aside stole my center. And I wonder if you know what it feels like to lose your center too.

I moved to the east side of the state and stayed with my Aunt Rhonda and my Uncle Rik. I was sure that Mom would miss me so much and that it would be enough to make her quit drinking. So I didn't unpack, for months and months. Boxes full, stacked in a corner waiting to move back home, waiting for her to change to save me, to save us, waiting to be worth coming for.

All sorts of folks from all sorts of backgrounds, experiences, and beliefs were gathered round Jesus one day, when He busted into a story about one lost sheep.[1] He said emphatically, "Suppose one of you has a hundred sheep and loses one of them. Doesn't he leave the ninety-nine in the open country and go after the lost sheep until he finds it?"[2] Jesus tells this story like it's a big "Duh." Like, of course you'd do whatever it took to go after the one. And yet, you and I haven't been worthy of showing up for. Our parent people couldn't or wouldn't get their act together to come for us. Our spouses didn't do the work to make it work. Our "good" friends let us go like we were one of many. Our shepherds, spiritual or otherwise, let us run away in the daylight, making no effort to come after us. I suppose what makes us feel the most lost is not that we wandered but that no one thought us worthy of pursuing.

I missed my mom something terrible. I missed her hugs. I missed hearing "I love you." I missed feeling known by the one who knew me most. I missed my friends, my team, my boyfriend. I missed my town. I missed the regulars at the café. I missed the random dogs wandering Main Street that would wag their tails at me like I was *their* kid. I missed the trails that had become a part of me.

I was so used to Roslyn, even the paths were my chums—I knew every bend, alley, pothole, pine tree, and lilac bush. I knew every house color and whose Aunt Sal lived where. I knew where to pick dandelions to blow wishes, and I knew the back way to the park. I knew the cracks in the sidewalks you couldn't roller-skate on. I knew that when Jan worked at the café, I could get leftover pie pastry baked with cinnamon and sugar. I knew that when Molly was in the kitchen, I should stay out. I knew when Tom worked at the theater, I could get extra gravy on my popcorn and when the first snow came, it was time to get out the sleds.

This move found no familiarity in its path.

No longer would the fresh Roslyn air waft into my bedroom window and put me to sleep. Never again would I hang my coat on the second hook in the hall. Gone were the snowy days of standing in front of our woodstove, letting it defrost my body and my mittens. I had to put down the orange phone I had used since I could dial to call numbers I knew by heart. The familiarly unremarkable might actually be what makes life remarkable. And what was familiar was no longer familiar. And what was home was never home again.

Eventually, I had to walk out of my aunt and uncle's basement and try to make a friend. I was going to die listening to melancholy '80s music, waiting for something to save me. I had tasted acceptance and friendship and a village and lost it because I needed rescue. And my need to be rescued might have made the likes of Jesus hop a fence and come running.

I started to find myself in the places that move you up the social ladder fastest—in trucks on high hills with boys pretending to care about me but only thinking about themselves. I drove drunk when I couldn't even walk. I would skip eating so I could get drunk faster. On prom night, I passed out on the toilet after puking. When I drank, I didn't feel pain, and not feeling felt like my cure.

I would get in conversations with Uncle Rik about Jesus. He didn't just talk about God, he lived grace. When I blew it and got caught sneaking out, getting wasted, and bald-faced lying about it, he looked at me, sad.

It wasn't the kind of pity-sad that only wants you to follow a set of rules because then you will be easier to deal with. It was the kind of sad that cared about where I was going with my life.

I remember asking Uncle Rikky once about his faith, "What if you're totally wrong about Jesus? What if it's all for nothing?"

He said, "Willy . . ." Secretly, I really liked that he had a special name for me. I was grateful that he swept me up and that he and his wife took me in when I needed it. I liked that he talked to me about what he cared about most.

What I didn't know then I know now. This Jesus my Uncle Rikky loved, He cares about lost sheep with everything He's got. He even said that when one lost sheep is found, it ought to be joyfully put on one's shoulders, brought home, and celebrated.[3]

A lot of us who've felt tossed aside, been dropped off miles from home, and waited years to be found so we could finally unpack those boxes—we think God doesn't care, doesn't see, doesn't come. I couldn't see it then, but I can now: When God comes to rescue us, He often uses people to do it. God sends His like-hearted people on rescue missions. We don't recognize it as God. But all those people you've run into—the sent ones who pointed you home, gave you a safe space to be, showed you your worth, took joy in your presence, gave you a nickname, and made sacrifices for your betterment—they are proof. God will move heaven and earth and leave whatever He has to in order to rescue you.

Having no idea Uncle Rik was sent to me by God, I listened closely to every word he said because he didn't just talk the talk. He picked me up and brought me home. I was more lost than I even knew and unwilling to let my heart unpack, but my uncle showed me I was worthy of family every single day.

Uncle Rikky responded to my question about his faith, "Willy, if I'm all wrong, I can't imagine living a better life than the one lived with Jesus."

But I wouldn't turn from *my* faith either. No, my faith was in myself. I wasn't a savior, but I was a survivor. I had faith that my strength had gotten me this far. I was certain God was nowhere to be found. What a no-show. My faith was in my need to be right about thinking people of faith were wrong, with their stiff ideals and their rigid rules. They were wrong about their white, middle-class Jesus and their fake efforts to act like they love. I had faith in my right and a Christian's wrong. And here my uncle had faith in being right *and* faith in being wrong.

So I had my eye on him. I watched his every move.

Like a hawk.

Because God knows, I needed rescue.

12

thirst traps

Not long ago, a woman with a trendy business suit and a designer purse, looking all put together, walked into the Collide office wanting to talk. She shared how much she resonated with my story. She talked about her childhood and how much pain her parents' addiction caused her. I asked about her life now. She showed me an Instagram-worthy picture of a beautiful family—a husband and three daughters. I said, "Wow, you guys look so happy."

"Yes, my family *looks* happy," she said. "But, what I haven't told you is that I have a . . . meth problem." I was floored. She had come to several of our Collide events, and after the first one, she got rid of all her drug paraphernalia. She was doing good and then COVID-19 hit, and she went back to the stuff. Two years later she had come to a Collide event again and then had gotten a tattoo of something we preached. She pulled up her sleeve and showed me the truth she never wanted to forget.

"Worthy of more."

Desperate for a change, she said, "I can't keep this up. I need help. I need healing. That's why I'm here. I know I can't keep doing the same things and expect different results."

This woman had collided with her wounded parents, and now she was wounding herself and her own children. It was like I was sitting with myself and my mother.

One night, Mom was sitting on the window seat looking out at the Roslyn ridge. Our living area above the café had a window-lined wall with an incredible view of the forest that surrounded our town, the trees that grew into forever—the ones my mom fought to keep alive with the people my friends whispered were "tree huggers."

Mom was staring out the window, holding a white café mug with its usual wine-stained brim. Her eyes were fixed, almost as though she was waiting, though for what, I wasn't sure.

I looked out the window too. On the ridge, a white cross lit up every night. In fact, it still does. Its presence always intrigued me. I didn't know the claim nor the controversy. I didn't know the truth nor the lies. I didn't know a Lord nor a Lord's story. But that there cross caught my eye, and I would wonder at it.

"What's wrong, Mama?"

She clutched the cup and took a sip. "It's Grandma Kathryn's birthday."

Grandma Kathryn passed away when I was two. She drank herself to death. Now, at five years old, I sat in my mother's grief as though I had inherited both their pain. This rich inheritance would pay for years to come.

In fact, I still get checks.

The cross lit up. It stared back at us—almost as though it were saying something. If only I had known what it said. We waited, not just that night, but always, for a love and a hope, a healing and a peace, to come and mend the pain that was passed from

my grandmother

to

my mother

to

me.

My Grandma Kathryn was a menagerie of things. She was gorgeous and creative, artistic and smart, unpredictable and spiritually curious. She visited churches, temples, and synagogues with my mom in tow, trying to experience a Divine Being she had a keen awareness of. She painted beautiful pieces, was an amazing cook, and loved the beach as much as I do. Kathryn lived a socialite life in Portland and married a successful businessman, my grandfather, who was preoccupied with his own ventures and adventures, leaving her deeply lonely. She often got sloppy drunk and things we can't talk about.

My mom always said her mother died from lack of love. I always thought that was just one alcoholic making an excuse for another. But over time, my own life changed my mind.

A dozen years later, I found myself trapped in my own efforts to get love. The summer after high school, I went to a house party with a guy from work. He had a crush on me, but it wasn't mutual. After getting boozed up, we started playing quarters. And I lost.

When you lose at quarters, you don't just lose quarters.

A guy I'd never met lured me into a back room. We lay on a bed in the dark, and I was puppeteered by his hands, the hard alcohol, and a deep desire to be loved. This wasn't the first nor the last time I'd get hurt trying to get love.

The guy who had invited me walked in and found me hooking up with his best friend. Enraged, he demanded I get my clothes on, and then he dragged me out of the room and shamed me in front of all his friends for being such a mess.

His angry disgust felt strangely familiar. All my life, my mother's partying had often led to some kind of repulsive behavior with a male houseguest that I had to endure. When I was in middle school, Mom fell in love with this odd, kind, imaginative, pirate-like jokester. I liked him sober, but his abuse of alcohol wrecked anything likable about him.

It felt as though I lost her entirely while she was with him. They would escape for the night, a weekend, and weeks, leaving me at home alone with the cats or a local troubled teen. Their escapades triggered an anger in me that slammed doors, threw things, and scorned them like children, all coming from a deep feeling of wanting control and having none.

One night in ninth grade, I woke up to Mom and her boyfriend drunk as skunks, doing things no kid should find their parent people doing. Enraged, I demanded she get her clothes on, and then I dragged her away from my room, shaming her in front of her boyfriend for being such a mess. Like the only adult in the room, I disrespectfully sent those two fools to her room so I could get some sleep. If you were my parent, you'd probably want to ground me. But it'd be kind of hard to do that when I'd already grounded you.

This wouldn't be the first nor the last time I'd get hurt while Mom was trying to get love.

Maybe my mom had been right about what killed my grandmother. Maybe she had turned to alcohol when she had lacked love. And had turned to love when she had drunk her fill of alcohol. All I really know is that I lacked love too, and it was starting to kill me just like it had started to kill my grandmother and my mother.

Some say the apple doesn't fall far from the tree. Some call it generational sin. I say wounds travel. They travel from your grandmother to your mother to you, and if you don't get healing, they will travel to your daughter and her daughter and *her* daughter.

Turns out, a lack of love *can* be the end of you.

Lack of love can find you doing things you said you would never do. You are becoming the very person you said you'd never become because you are chasing love and you can't run fast enough to catch it. But the very things you are doing to catch that love are the very things that make you feel more and more unlovable.

If only I had known I was already loved.

College looked like story after story of drunken stupors, drinking and driving, hiding from the cops, getting written up, skipping class, passing out, alcohol poisoning, sloppy hookups, and shame hangovers. I was majoring in wounding people and minoring in stupidity. And I was beginning to walk a strangely familiar path. I had seen where this trail leads. I just hadn't been the one walking it . . . until now.

From quarters guy

to

guy up on a hill in a truck

to

guy I felt sorry for

to

guy in the dorms

to

guy I met on the dance floor

to

guy I dumped that I loved too much.

And then to SchmuckFaceBibleBoy. The day after we had sex, he showed up to my dorm room crying remorsefully, "I am sorry. What

I did was wrong, and I need to tell you about Jesus." And that was when he handed me my very first Bible. The only other time I'd been given one was by some Bible-thumpers on campus, and I'd thrown that one back. This guy was the one who actually deserved a Bible thrown in his face. What a nimrod.

I didn't like Christians and certainly wasn't looking to be one. For years, I made fun of God's people. I had no desire to get thorn tats and listen to lame music about angels and bloody lambs. Nothing in me wanted to live a dreadfully uptight life. How could I ever say yes to monogamy and church organs? I would never like potluck casseroles. And Sundays were for nursing hangovers. This hippie girl raised by a strong female activist was not going to go down the Jesus path without a good fight.

At some point in college, I picked up the black book that had been sitting on my shelf since SchmuckFace gave it to me. I started reading page 1. "In the beginning . . ." It seemed like things were awesome until the apple, and then they got really screwed up. Like things were perfect and then Adam, the first father, blew it, and his sons were ruined, and they ruined their sons, and everything was a bloody, wounded mess with orphans and anger and widows and war, and I bet there were even sad girls getting sloppy drunk to numb the pain, sleeping with men just like their fathers.

I put the book back on the shelf . . .

I ended up in a hotel room one night, desperate for rescue. Desperate, not like so many times before, but worse, like my life was accumulating a brokenness that I couldn't make go away. I couldn't numb it. I couldn't find a love to satiate it. I couldn't save myself from my life and its overwhelming, toppling, crushing weight.

Jesus collided with a woman in John 4 who might have understood this feeling of accumulating brokenness, shame, and despair.[1] She was thirsty as could be and wouldn't you know it, Jesus showed up at her well. But isn't this where God meets us? The apple might not fall far from the tree, but God doesn't fall far from the apple. I mean let's be real. As soon as Adam and Eve took a bite of that thing, it was like God showed up mid-crunch. No sooner did Adam and Eve start hiding in their shame than God was found looking for them. This woman was at a well at an hour when no one else went. But there was Jesus waiting for her.

God is a God who shows up in the room where you are being puppeteered. He shows up and speaks to you through a cross when all you feel like doing is drinking to grieve your dead alcoholic mother. God shows up right where He knows you will be—because you always go there. And there you are, predictable as can be, like a well-worn path carried you to the same ol' watering hole that will be just another thirst trap. And He meets you there because He wants more for you than what your wounded history offers.

Jesus asked the woman for some water, which was crazy. And she knew it. She was a Samaritan, and Samaritans were considered less-than and morally far from God, forbidden to enter the inner courts of the Temple. Plus, as a woman, she was devalued, discounted, and deemed a second-class citizen. For Jesus to engage the likes of her was unheard of.

And here she was, drawing water, because she was so very thirsty. Jesus offered her something for her thirst. "Living water," He called it.[2] She missed His point. She got practical and He got spiritual. They bantered back and forth, and Jesus suggested that if she drank the water He gave, she would never thirst.

She said, "Give me the water so I won't be thirsty and have to keep coming back here." Jesus responded, "Go get your husband." And she said, "I don't have a husband." And He said "You're right . . . You've had five husbands, and the man you're with now is not your husband."

Jesus wasn't shaming her. Jesus was helping her recognize a pattern in her life that was not working.

Husband

to

husband

to

husband

to

husband

to

husband

to

new guy.

Look, no one wants to hear, "There's a trend in your life that's not working." But if we don't see the pattern, we will keep biting the apple we never wanted to, keep drinking the promise of a fulfillment that never fills, keep waking up in beds we wish were ours, keep becoming more and more like the person we never wanted to be.

Jesus knows we have to see our own tendency to drink from wells that make us sick. He allows us to see it, to feel it, to taste it. He knows we have to recognize our brokenness before we will want to become more whole. After all, it is only when we sip cup after cup after cup and none of it really takes the pain away, but only causes more, that we begin to consider there might be something else that can actually satisfy.

I needed healing in a wholly desperate way, and I knew it. I knew it that night in the hotel room like that girl at the well probably knew it. I knew it like Jesus Himself must have been standing in room 317 watching me come undone.

I got to the terrifying edge of myself. And there I was, dangling. I felt as alone as I have ever felt. I knew I needed more than me. But I didn't believe in more. I hadn't believed there was a God, a Creator, a Lord. I not only *didn't* believe that, I hadn't *wanted* to.

I was sure that even if I called out for rescue, this God, if He were real, would leave me in my want because somehow I deserved all this pain. I assumed God would not help me in my brokenness. I have come to realize that I share that assumption with many others. Maybe even you.

I wanted to be found by God for the first time in my life, but I was sure He wouldn't want anything to do with the likes of me. But I needed God like I needed breath, like I needed water, like I needed healing, like I needed love. So I did something I had never done. I called out to the walls, to the echoes, to the atmosphere. I cried out, hoping I was not alone, afraid for what it might mean if I was. *Is there anyyyyone who caaaan hellllp me? Godddd, if You are real, can You help me?*

This was my first conversation with God.

I broke to such a degree that I actually called out to a God I didn't know was there. I so clearly saw that lack of love would be the end of me. I put down the coffee mug with the wine-stained brim. I could no longer be my own cure, no longer be my own rescue, no longer perpetuate the pattern I was born into. And this breaking would be what broke the messy, destructive, wounded pattern I had inherited.

Our wounded patterns are not a surprise to Jesus. He knew how the woman at the well got there. He knew why she was so parched. So what did He do? He offered Himself. That might sound woo-woo. It might sound so impractical that you are rolling your eyes. But what else can quench our thirst? Jesus offered this woman what He offers us, saying, "When you're thirsty, come to Me instead of all the other things you try again and again. I will satisfy."

This woman had her first conversation with Jesus, and she was impacted so much that she left her water jar and ran into town! Leaving your water jar looks different for all of us, but it always looks like recognizing that what you have been doing isn't working and maybe, just maybe, it's time to do something entirely different.

This woman left what she once used to fill her thirst and ran to share her collision-with-Jesus story with her city. "Come and see," she said, and they all came running to collide with Jesus. She impacted the very people who once might have judged, shamed, and disrespected her. Did you know this woman with the long list of husbands is considered one of the first evangelists? She might have thought her story was about losing at quarters, losing at relationships, losing at life, but when Jesus got ahold of her story of brokenness, He purposed it for healing.

Sitting in the Collide office, I looked at the mom on meth, wanting nothing more than for her to get better for herself and for her kids. I said, "I am about to say something to you that I hope you hear in love. I am saying it because we get each other's stories. If you keep this up, your kids will feel the way *you* have felt your entire life. They will feel like they weren't enough for you to choose them over this addiction. They will feel unworthy, and they, too, will need to numb the pain your addiction caused."

I hoped somehow God could use me to create an indelible moment, one where she walked out different than she walked in. "You have an opportunity *right now* to change the trajectory of your life and your kids' lives," I said. That day she set down meth and picked up Jesus and counseling and her very first Bible. I handed it to her, knowing the words would change her life, just like they changed mine.

The words on her arm would soon be written on her heart. The worth Jesus sees in her, He has always seen in her. And His love for her didn't show up for the first time on the day she received it. He's been chasing her down since day one, trying to tattoo His love on her life. She needed to know what we all need to know: A new story is possible.

Take it from me, an old get-around girl: Once God gets ahold of your story, there's no telling what He will do. He can take all your pain, all your regret, all your big, bad mistakes, all the generational waywardness passed down to you, all the patterns you keep repeating—He can take all of it and write a different story than the one you inherited. And that, my friend, will change your children's story and their children's story. So put down the cup, call out to the walls, collide with the One who offers not a cheap, wine-stained fix, but His very self.

Come and see . . .

13

if you hads

I collided into a blind man.

With my car.

As soon as I felt the impact, I looked up and saw his cane tapping my hood.

Frazzled, with my kid in the back seat, music still blaring, and a window that wouldn't roll down, I started panic sweating. By the time I could collect myself, he had taken his foot out from under the front tire, made his way around my car, and gotten quite a ways down the sidewalk. "Sorrrrrrrry!" I yelled, trying to reach him with an apology.

He replied like it happens every day, "That's ohhhhkay." I felt terrible. Lucky for me, he couldn't take down my license plate.

Sometimes in life, the thing we wish to see most, we don't see at all. This is how it was for Mary and Martha in John 11.[1] Life was going along just fine and *Boom!* Something unexpected hit them. Their brother Lazarus became deathly ill. They sent word to Jesus, saying, "Lord, the one you love is sick."[2] But Jesus refused to show up.

All these sisters wanted was to see God show up with a blessing, a rescue, a healing. They wanted to see God bring the same power He brought to the Red Sea, the leper, the storm. But to our collective dismay, Jesus didn't run to their rescue. This is the Jesus we don't like. This is the Jesus who disappoints us. The One who doesn't do what we want Him to.

Jesus waited two days and said to His disciples, "This sickness will not end in death . . . it is for God's glory."[3] Now I don't know about you, but the idea of bringing God glory in exchange for someone I love doesn't make me wanna slap on a fish tat and follow Jesus wherever He goes. The entire community showed up for these women, but not Jesus. This must have been the longest forty-eight hours of Mary's and Martha's lives. The Bible straight up says Jesus *loved* Martha, Mary, and Lazarus. As backward as it feels, Love doesn't always show up the way we expect it to.

It was a common Jewish belief that there was no hope once a person had been dead longer than four days. The body would have had obvious decay, and the soul would have departed. By the time Jesus rolled in, Lazarus was considered a "four-day man."[4]

Jesus often shows up right when we think it's game over.

Martha went to meet Jesus, and you can hear her disappointment. She said, "If you had been here, my brother would not have died."[5] Her grief was real, but so was her faith. For some crazy reason she was still holding on to the belief that Jesus was good. He assured her that her brother would rise, and then He laid out a huge claim: "I am the resurrection and the life. The one who believes in me will live, even though they die; and whoever lives by believing in me will never die. Do you believe this?"[6]

Martha's brother was dead. She was disappointed and angry. Here she was smack-dab in the chapter of her story she never wanted written, and yet she said, "Yes, Lord . . . I believe that you are the Messiah, the Son of God." Martha ran to get her sister, and Mary came to Jesus, fell at his feet, and said, "Lord, if you had been here, my brother would not have died."[7]

Both Martha and Mary brought their "if You hads" to Jesus. And you know what? I think we need to bring ours to Him too.

If You had healed them.

If You had protected me as a kid.

If You had stopped my dad from leaving.

If You had stopped the abuse.

If You had brought justice.

If You had only looked after, been near, shown up.

My biggest hang-up with God echoed Martha's and Mary's: *Where were You when I needed You?*

By the time I was a junior in college, life caught up with me. I broke down and ended up withdrawing from my classes. I couldn't carry the pain, the shame, the secrets. I couldn't carry a relationship, a grade, a self-esteem.

I could no longer carry the job of rescuing me.

After my *If You're real, God, I need help* prayer in the hotel room, God started stalking me. I have often heard people describe God as the Hound of Heaven, and boy, did He chase after me. My hairdresser was Christian, my coworkers were Christian. Heck, my dog was probably Christian. I had no idea how I had let such characters sneak into my story. I hadn't ever given God the time of day, let alone His people.

I ended up pulling that black book off the shelf again. Its words will pierce any open heart. And my heart was as open as a heart in need of surgery would be. I figured if the words in this book were His words, the words of the One who made everything, the One who sculpted me in my mother's womb . . . what would He say to me about this mess everyone has all over them? What would He say about our pain? How was He going to rescue us?

It was with this posture that I would eventually give Jesus a chance.

Estranged from my dad, an ocean away from my mom, having lost my college squad, and in a housing situation surrounded by cokeheads, I knew I needed to pack fast. I had done it before; I could do it again.

It's often in the low places that the Divine is found, colliding with us in ways we could never imagine but so desperately need. But right before that, all we can see is our car packed up with all our belongings and no place to call home. We might not be looking for something God-smacked. We might just be looking for a new address. And friend, it's usually in this kind of place that we find what we aren't looking for.

And maybe what I am about to tell you is the whole reason I ever ended up with "Sorry we had sex, here's a Bible" boy. So get ready for a "my cousin married their cousin, whose dog married that dog's cousin" story . . .

The week I had to move out, SchmuckFaceBibleBoy's mom went to visit his ex-wife, who was house-sitting for her friend Cindy. While they were chatting, the tenant from the basement apartment came up and dropped off her "I'm moving out" notice. Schmucky's mom knew that I needed a place to live, and God forbid I move in with her son, so she got the landlord's number from her ex-daughter-in-law to give to me, the wayward, slutty girlfriend. I warned you it would be confusing. But that's what God stories are like. God stories are like your boyfriend's ex-wife's friend ends up being the thing that changes your life.

This is how I met Cindy Aubert, a woman just bold enough that I couldn't help but give her brand of crazy Christian a listen. Cindy said I could move into her basement *but* I couldn't have boys overnight *and* I couldn't party. I had never heard of anything more archaic. I moved in with the idea that I would only *temporarily* not have sex or drink.

The Aubert's living room might have been the closest thing to the café that I had experienced since I lived in Roslyn. All sorts of characters sat at Cindy's table: people fresh out of rehab, newly divorced people broken as heck, and churchy chicks who spoke a language I didn't understand. Cindy fed people, poured oil on people, and prayed over people the kind of prayers that give you the goosies. She belly laughed with you one minute, and the next she looked you straight in the eye and told you the hard truth. Plus, she made a mean garlic bread.

Cindy welcomed me into her days, her people, and her heart. When she called me out, I knew it was because she loved me. She was off-puttingly certain but also broken enough that I could relate to her redemption story because I needed one too. I could see in Cindy struggle, hunger, and pain, but I could also see Jesus.

Cindy invited me to share my story, and as I did, it was like I was hearing it for the first time. I had never felt like I had permission to give my own experience oxygen. And here I was, breathing.

Cindy kept pointing my story to Jesus' story. And I pushed back: "But where was He when I needed Him?" She kept showing up, holding space for my pain and grief. Each time I collided with Cindy, I felt like the divine needle and thread were sewing stitches in the places I needed mending most.

Around this time, I started meeting with a counselor who turned out to be Christian too. Karolyn could see my deep desire to understand where God was when I had needed Him. Every week I walked out of our sessions wanting it to be the next week already. I was unloading years of story, including my "if You hads."

During one session, Karolyn asked me to travel back and think of a difficult moment as a little girl. I got a picture right away. There was no belligerent drunk man. No group of adults trying to learn the violin at 2 a.m. on a school night. No mirror with straws and coke on the dining room table. The first thing I pictured seemed so "ordinary." Ten-year-old me was sitting on our tattered old plum velvet chair, all by myself, wanting *not* to be. The loneliness was speaking. It said to me what it still does, *You deserve to be alone*.

The counselor asked me to invite Jesus to sit with me on that chair. Why would someone willingly ask God to sit in their pain? I couldn't do it.

Here's the beautiful thing about that collision with Mary and Martha: Jesus could have said, "Look, ladies, you are merely two of the gazillion people on the planet who need Me." But He didn't. Jesus not only handled their pain, but He felt their feels. The Bible says, "Jesus wept."[8] This might be the most understated Scripture ever. A God who feels, emotes, and *empathizes* with us? Sit and ponder that for a lifetime.

While God was stalking me, I kept reading the Bible. I remember crashing the Aubert's Bible study group. I felt like a foreigner around Christians, but I wanted answers for my one million questions. "Why does God allow suffering? Why do you think Jesus is God, the Savior, the answer to all our freaking problems?" No kidding, I even asked, "What if there are aliens, what would that mean about Jesus?" I mean, I think I annoyingly covered all the bases.

To my surprise, Jesus partied with sinners, turned water into the best Bordeaux you've ever had, fed the hungry, took care of the poor, told religiously stuffy people to lose their judgmental snobbery, called

His followers to take care of widows and orphans, and gave His life for yours and mine. I started to think, *If this is what God is like, I want more of Him*, reluctantly, but for real.

After months of my constant questions, Steve Aubert leveled with me. He could see I didn't like my story. I wanted it to write differently, and if it had, then maybe I would believe there was a God. With a little bit of teasing and a lot of love, Steve said, "Willow, at some point it comes down to faith." Ultimately, he was inviting me to trust God as the Author of my story, to believe that God can take all these wounded, broken chapters and write better ones. To stop trying to make sense of my pain and instead look to the Healer for a new future. Steve invited me, and I invite you, into the crazy idea of having faith in a God, a story, a healing that we can't see yet.

I finally invited Jesus to go back and sit with ten-year-old me on that tattered plum velvet chair. I was sitting there alone, picking my nails until they were bloody, some already gone. I was ashamed, inducing a self-harm I could not hide. My cat Bennie crawled up in my lap, but what I really wanted was Mom home. I cried and cried, reliving that sorrow. And Jesus wept with me. I let every last disappointment come flooding out. I told Him how let down I felt by Him.

Jesus shared my sadness. He stood close, whispering over me what I was intended to have, what I deserved, what I was worthy of. He spoke truth into all the lies loneliness had told that little girl. And slowly, as Jesus held space for my pain, I allowed Him to pick me up and hold me. I plopped up in Jesus' embrace and wept with Him for the brokenness of it all.

On that day and so many others after it, I have had to invite Jesus into my sorrow. He is called a Man of Many Sorrows.[9] Jesus understands suffering. In fact, it is why He came to crash into and collide with humanity—because we suffer.

If anyone is able to sit in your wounds, your loneliness, your grief, your chair . . . it's Jesus. He can handle all of your "if You hads." And honestly, for some of us, this is where we have to start with Jesus right now. We can't start with an "I believe in You." We can't fake the amens. We have to start with a "Where were You, God?! All I wanted was to see You."

You might have to pull a Martha and Mary and tell Jesus you feel like He failed you. It's in this raw, uncensored honesty with God that our pain and His healing intersect. The day I got *this* real with Jesus, Jesus became real to me. In my brutally honest, plainspoken truth, I spared Him no pain. I was met with His love and His presence in a way that began stitching up a lifetime of open wounds. And friend, I don't think I could have arrived at this kind of trust and closeness with Jesus had I held him at a distance from my ugly grief.

After God met me on that chair, I began to see that God shows up—in the Cindys, the Steves, and the Karolyns. Cindy was right: Our story and pain matter, and making space for them makes space for Jesus. Steve was right: Trusting God to be the Author of our whole story helps us to see the healing we can't yet in the most difficult chapters. God will usher in good out of hard, healing out of pain, redemption out of brokenness, and resurrection out of death. He is writing a really good story out of being two days late and what seems like twenty years overdue. Karolyn was right too: Our healing hangs on the need to allow Jesus to go back to where we first picked up the pain.

The more we invite Jesus into our "if You hads," the more we will be met by the One who resurrects healing chapters out of wounded ones. The most incredible, life-giving, hope-bringing turn of events was about to happen to Mary and Martha . . . and their dead brother. But first, they had to wait for Jesus. Let's allow Jesus to meet us like He met them.

We want to fast-forward to the happy part, but when we ignore our own pain, it never actually goes away. We want to pretend we're good with God, but we won't *be* good with God if we just pretend. True healing requires we bring it all to God—even the pain we started believing He is responsible for. True healing requires us to grieve with God. And sometimes that even looks like grieving God *with* God—that is, with our wrong beliefs about Him.

Rather than skipping to the happily-ever-after part and not being happy after all, let us run toward Jesus. Let's fall at His feet, not in a grand gesture but in the sloppy, messy, snot-wiping cryfest of our grief. Let's be real because we only want a Jesus who is real. And if *He* is real, He can handle when *we* are. Jesus can heal and mend and stitch us back up, but we have to let Him into the pain. Let's not jump to the resurrection chapter. We've been skipping ahead for way too long. Instead, let's meet Jesus on the chair.

14

reckless

There were stars like you've never seen in Roslyn, but there were also trees older than you and your dad put together. There were people, and there were dogs, lotsa dogs. There was freedom, and nothing kept you from exploring it. I think growing up in Roslyn shaped me in ways I will never quite grasp. There was nothing to do and everything to do all at once. There was no superstore, no mall, no arcade, no bowling alley. You had to get inventive and come up with your own way to fill a Saturday.

If Mom was busy and I was bored, I'd roam the streets. My cousin Andrea and I would make chamomile tea from the herbs we picked on her dirty gravel driveway. I would run up the slag piles left over from the old mines just so I could run back down. I would pick tansy, a small, hardy yellow flower that grew like weeds in Roslyn, and on my way to almost anywhere, I would recite "He loves me, he loves me not," thinking of my latest crush. I had lots of crushes: boys I chased, boys I hoped would take notice of me, and boys that never did. The ones I wanted to like me didn't, and the ones I didn't did. That theme carried on into my twenties, and maybe you can relate.

Maybe it was my raggedy short hair and the fact that I couldn't change it until I was old enough to say heck no to a hairdresser. Maybe it was because I liked to catch tadpoles and play basketball. I don't know why so many boys liked Jenny and Kristi instead of me. My fate in love was always determined by which line of the song fell on the last tansy popped off the stem.

On my way home one day, I ran smack-dab into a boy on the Fifth Street alley. We had a wounded collision, right there with the garter snakes and the dust as our witnesses. He said with vengeance, "Where is yourrrr daaaad?" I was seven—no one had ever asked me this question. And I wasn't sure I knew the answer. Just thinking about the facts made me feel sad but also accused, like I had done something wrong. My volume turned sheepish and stuttery, "He . . . uh . . . he lives far away."

This kid decided to let me in on the truth: "Your dad doesn't love you. If he did, he'd live with you . . . but he doesn't, soooo . . ." He said these words angrily, as if he wanted me to know not only just how unloved I was but also how absolutely true it was. I wanted to bring something to the harsh debate, but I could not prove him wrong.

The news stunned me only because someone said it. Out. Loud. Everything now made sense. It set me straight about who I was and who I wasn't. I kept walking with my tansies, singing the song I normally sang with a boy in mind. But this time the boy was my father.

He loves me . . .

He loves me not . . .

He loves me . . .

Popping the blooms off one by one until I came to the last one . . .

He loves me not.

Something in me broke that day. It was almost formulaic, like math. Two minus one equals one. If your dad loved you, he would be with you. He isn't with you, so he doesn't love you. Therefore, there's something about you that makes you unlovable.

Often the belief you and I attach to brokenness in relationship is *I would be loved IF*________. You are loved IF your dad lives with you. You are a good little girl IF you follow all the rules. God will answer your prayers IF you do all the right things. Your spouse will stay with you IF you stay attractive. Your boyfriend won't move on IF you have sex. Your community will accept you IF you believe what they believe and hate all the same people they hate. Your parents will brag about you IF they are proud of your behavior, and they'll put you in a corner IF they aren't.

We have all loved and been loved IF. All this conditional loving has helped us develop a conditional theology, one in which we decide God loves *us* IF and God loves *others* IF. God loves them IF they check all the boxes, IF they believe all the right things, IF they behave the way we think they should. IF they, IF they, IF they.

There is a collision in Luke 15 where Jesus challenged our concept of conditional love.[1] Jesus was at a party, and while He was reaching for more little smokies, some religious folk piped up with disdain for the people He was hanging with at this shindig.

Imagine how the *sinners* felt hearing this. Would Jesus love them, or would He agree that they weren't worthy of coming home for? You can almost hear the record scratch and the music stop. The whole party was waiting to see how Jesus would respond. And then He busted into one of the most beautiful stories you've ever heard.

He told the story of the prodigal son who demanded his father give him his inheritance early. In Jewish culture, this would have been shocking. The people eating charcuterie would have gasped. They would have choked on the olives in their martinis. Inheritance was a huge deal. There was law and ritual and honor and legacy all wrapped up in it. And it was never given away until the end of one's life. This was like the son saying, "I wish you were dead."

Everyone would have expected the father to give the son what he deserved—punishment, lectures, disinheritance—anything but honor for this ungrateful brat. But the father gave him his inheritance.

The son took off and lived *la vida loca*: champagne, caviar, yachts, Range Rovers, girls here, girls there, a strip club one night, a casino the next. He spent his inheritance on what the Bible calls "wild living." This son didn't get the nickname "prodigal" for nothing. The word means spending freely and recklessly or being wastefully extravagant.[2] This kid blew it *all.*

If this wasn't bad enough, an economic depression hit. People were being laid off, they were losing their houses, the food bank line was longer than ever, theft was surging, depravity was intensifying, and this kid found himself feeding pigs for a job. He got so hungry he longed to eat the pigs' food.

Now, you have to hear this story like those at the party heard it. Pigs were abhorred by Jewish people. You wouldn't even come into contact with one, ever, no matter how desperate you got.[3]

The Bible says that right there with pig slop all over him, this young man "came to his senses."[4] We have to know how important this is. God uses even the pig slop. It wasn't the father's ranting, the father's "You should be ashamed of yourself," or the father's passive-aggressive texts that woke this kid up. It was the low place.

Right there at rock bottom, the prodigal son remembered his father—his years of sacrifice, teaching, hard work, grace, love, truth, care, and investment. Sometimes we remember the character of a parent when we're surrounded by pigs. Sometimes we remember we're the child of a King when we've become the servant of sin. Sometimes we remember we miss home when we're about as far away from it as we can be.

This guy said to himself, "I will set out and go back to my father and say to him: Father, I have sinned against heaven and against you. I am no longer worthy to be called your son; make me like one of your hired servants."[5] And you can picture him, right? Like a little girl poppin' tops off tansies . . .

He loves me . . .

He loves me not . . .

But this son didn't have to go far. In one of the most moving verses in the Bible, we read, "While he was still a long way off, his father saw him and was filled with compassion for him; he ran to his son, threw his arms around him and kissed him."[6] The son was embraced with . . .

He loves me . . .

He loves me . . .

He loves me . . .

Perhaps what gets me most is that the father was probably waiting for his kid on that hill every single day. Imagine holding on to hope and falling apart in anguish all at the same time. Imagine not sleeping at night, worried sick. Imagine waiting every day for a change, for a sign of hope, for their heart to return to yours. Maybe you don't have to imagine. Maybe you know this feeling all too well.

As soon as the father saw the son coming, he sprinted toward his boy. He hugged the heck out of his kid who was covered in pig slop.

He called his staff and said, "Bring the best robe. He is my son. I am his father. Put the family signet ring on him to seal it. Give the boy shoes. Bring the best food. Let's celebrate! My dead son is alive! He was lost and is found!"

The father didn't lay out any conditions for the son to come back home. He didn't list all the ways he had been hurt. He didn't check how genuine the son's sorry was. The father didn't say, "Go prove you've changed and then come back and show me."

And the prodigal son? He didn't pay back what he had wasted. He didn't build back trust in the family. The son didn't even promise he would change.

The older brother showed up and was confused and angry. He had done all the right things, and his dad was celebrating all the *wrong* things? He was like we might be: "Really?! You're just gonna let this loser come prancing back?" The critical brother sounded exactly like the religious mutterers at the party where Jesus told the story.

Above all other things for the father was the son coming home. It's not that the father agreed with the son's attitude, behavior, or sin. It's not that the father didn't care about what the son believed, valued, or worshiped. But there is a difference between agreement and love. You don't have to agree to have relationship, but you do have to love. And maybe we need to be reminded of this more than we ever have.

Relationship seemed to be primary for the father. He cared more about the son than the son's mistakes, more about the son than the son's track record, more about the son than the son's alignment with his own beliefs, more about the son than the son's admission of sin. Our IF list often seems to be more about the sorry, the admission of guilt, the do-better plan, the proof of change, the "I agrees," and the "I won't do it agains." But not the Father's.

The Father wants us home more than He wants us perfect.

This is mind-blowing to me. This kind of love scares us. And it should. This is a reckless way to love. Some sinner's pig slop might get all over you. A celebration party over a disgraceful son might make you look like a fool. Your lenience could send the wrong message. Your wiping away of consequences could dilute the truth. You could get hurt by someone you love again. This is reckless.

We want a love that feels less risky.

You think this is a story about a prodigal son who is reckless in his sin. But it's not. This is a story about a prodigal Father who is reckless in His love. You think it's a story about someone else who is lost, but like the older brother, the lost one might just be you.

Remember the entire reason Jesus told this story? Some religious folk were judging Jesus for hanging out with sinners. The last thing these people far from their Father needed was to run into another mean boy reminding them of what they already feared might be true. Jesus responded with all the passion, compassion, and grace He had. This story was Jesus' full heart on display. In fact, some call it the gospel within the gospel.

We have a God who loves recklessly. Not long after telling this story, He would take all the mess, wrongdoing, waywardness, betrayal, inheritance demanding, grace manipulating, wild living, and sin on Himself. But for now, He would keep showing the runaways that they could always come home.

When I finally realized I had a Father who loved me so much that all He wanted was to be at home with me, I was overcome. After years of searching, at twenty-one years old, I came to my senses. You should have seen it.

I was sitting uncomfortably in the back room of a church that was giving 1995 Pentecostal mom vibes. I normally wouldn't have been caught dead in this kind of crowd, but because Cindy invited me, I went. So here I was in a room full of church chicks, and one of the women questioned me in front of everyone, "What are you waiting for?"

I needed that moment. I knew I wanted God in my life. I wanted Him more than any love or pleasure, more than anything I had ever drunk to quench my thirst and make me feel loved. I wanted Him to stay with me because He wanted to.

As soon as I expressed that I wanted God, about twenty sweet church ladies began praying over me. I could see my hands extending toward my Father in wild abandon. All the pain, confusion, questions and doubt, longing and grief, all the pig slop, my entire broken heart, and every road I walked that broke it, I placed in God's hands. I found the place I had wanted to belong my whole life . . . Home.

These women started praying in tongues and praying that I would too. But it wasn't happening. It freaked me right out. I wondered if I should fake them out or wait them out. I decided that if God was real, I would be too.

I ran out like a scary religious monster was chasing me, not sure if I would set foot in God's house again. That night I went to a party and got loaded, as was my usual recreational sport. It wasn't like I immediately traded my hobby in for scrapbooking the day I decided to follow Jesus.

It's not as easy as it looks to surrender your life, your ideals, your dreams, and your Friday nights. As much as some religious people want life change to be instantaneous, it often isn't. A life transformed requires time well spent with the One who does the transforming. The need for change over months, years, or decades does not mean

God is not real any more than it means that the still-sinning sinner's conversion isn't real.

My Lutheran friend Kristi, who never went to church but wore a cross and talked about her religion as though it was very important to her, was at the same party. Sloshed and slurring with genuine excitement, I said to her, "Guess whuuuut I did todaaaay? I gave my life to Jeeeesus." We boomed beer bottles, said, "Cheers!" and hugged. I went back downstairs and danced on the coffee table. But the me that was drunk dancing was different, and though no one else knew it, I did.

For some crazy reason, the next Sunday I drove by myself to a church. I sat in my car, afraid I might experience something else that made me feel Christian-creepy, and said in what I suppose you can call a prayer, *God, if this is where You want me, help me to know.*

I walked in and was overwhelmed by a sense of belonging. It wasn't the cookies. It definitely wasn't the coffee. I don't remember the sermon. Maybe it was the ex-heroin addict who ran into Jesus, got clean, and was bringing along others who needed the same power for their addiction. Maybe it was the pastor who talked about his past without covering it up. Maybe it was the businessman who found a place to drop his head in despair as he laid down his bankruptcy and picked up Jesus. It was the stories of lives that needed changing that made me feel like I belonged. This church felt like a place where you could open yourself up to the Love you needed, and that Love could change you into who you were made to become. It felt like I might have found a village again. I wanted my commitment to Jesus to feel authentic, so to my own surprise, I filled out one of those cheesy church cards and checked the box for *I give my life to Christ.*

The next week I was checking groceries to pay for my Long Island iced teas. I saw a lady standing behind me, so I said, "Can I help you?"

In a British accent, she said, "I knew you when you were a little girl, and I need to meet you for coffee."

Pam and I met the next week. She said her job was to go through the communication cards at the church I had randomly walked into. She came across my name and saw that I had given my life to Christ. She was floored and knew there couldn't be another person by that name.

She said, "I used to see you playing on the streets of Roslyn when you were little, and God told me to pray for you because you were hurting and you were going to need Him." She began to weep. "I prayed for you for *years*, and here you are, decades later, all the way across the state, and you walked into *my* church and gave your life to Christ. God has answered my prayers."

After a lifetime of hoping someone would come for me, I began weeping. My Father had been pursuing me all along.

He had waited on the hill every single day. He'd walked down every road. He called in the prayer warriors. He pursued me, chased me, hounded me, stalked me. He endured pig slop, hatred, cursing, and doubt, and He had patience for ignorance, selfishness, recklessness, and demands. He had broken through generational wounds, trauma, dysfunction, baggage, mindsets, misunderstanding, and battles to get me. And He does the same for you.

You and I are always wanted home. There is nothing—must I say it again?—there is *nothing* that makes this Father not want to be at home with you.

He loves you.

He loves you.

He loves you.

He loves you.

15

the over and over again

The year before I found Jesus, I was full of hatred and blame, avoiding Dad like the plague. I was no longer speaking to him, and in the trenches of my silence, he traveled hours out of his way to show up on my doorstep unexpectedly. I hid behind the curtain of my second-story window, watching him knock over and over again.

He continued to beat down the door of my life, and I refused to give in. I didn't have even a small desire to forgive my dad. I wanted him to suffer in his own regret, sit in his sorry, and never have the privilege of my presence again. I wanted him to hurt the way he had hurt me.

I was bitter as all get-out. *Why did you leave me when you left her? Why didn't you protect me when you knew I needed it? Why didn't you come when you could have? What was so important that your kid wasn't? You were choosing you. You never chose me. And now you want to?*

Looking down on him, with a lifetime of bitterness welling up, I spoke words he could not hear,

It's

a little

too

late.

My dad could have his blank pages, and I would hand him more by not forgiving him. We would have no words, no experiences, no memories, no relationship. He could have what he deserved, and I would make sure he knew *he chose it.*

Within a year of my dad knocking on my door, so did Jesus. I quickly learned I was called to forgive as He forgives. In fact, one of the first challenges Jesus handed me when I handed Him my life was to walk toward forgiveness with my dad. And when I say walk toward it, I mean just that. Some of us have been hurt so badly that forgiveness feels like a miracle, like an impossibility, like a million miles away. So we have to turn in its direction, taking one step at a time.

When Peter collided with Jesus in Matthew 18, he asked, "Lord, how many times shall I forgive my brother or sister who sins against me? Up to seven times?"[1] We read this story like Peter was striking up a theological discussion for the sake of conversation. But I'm convinced this was way more than that. Peter was no different than you and me. He probably had his own wounded collisions that left him angry and resentful. I believe Peter asked this question from a place of pain and an authentic inability to see how he could forgive the person who had caused it.

The Greek word used for *forgive* actually means to "send away" or to "let go."[2] Peter was asking, "How often do I let go of an offense when someone I love keeps hurting me?" It's the same question we ask. Maybe we just use different words:

"How many times do I let them off the hook when they know better?"

"You can only put up with so much, and then you just have to set your limits, right?"

"They'll never change, so why bother trying to forgive?"

"How much pain do I have to endure before I can walk away?"

Peter was wrestling. He wanted to know when he could just close the door on a difficult relationship and keep it closed. When Peter suggested forgiving someone seven times, he was thinking that's over-the-top gracious. Some rabbis limited forgiveness to three times. So, when your dad doesn't show up to your first day of kindergarten, and then he doesn't show up for your sixth birthday, and then he doesn't make it to your first basketball game . . . you can blank-page him. You can decide to no longer call him Dad, because dads show up. You can close the door, and no matter how hard he pounds on it, you can leave it locked and watch him suffer for all the ways *you* had to.

Jesus met Peter in his pain, but He didn't respond the way Peter expected. Jesus throws us all off with these words: "No, not seven times . . . but seventy times seven!"[3] This doesn't mean 490 times, you little math wizard, you. This is a Jewish phrase about never holding grudges. Some translators have tried to make sense of it by saying, "seven times and then again and again until you can't count."[4] Who can put up with that many offenses? But that's what Jesus was getting at. Theologian Warren Wiersbe says, "By the time we have forgiven a brother that many times, we are in the habit of forgiving."[5] We are not to put limits on our forgiveness, but to forgive so much, so often, that it's our go-to. It's on repeat. How many times? Over and over and over again.

Jesus told Peter a story to describe the Kingdom of God, the way life looks when God rules it.[6] He said it's like a king who called in a guy who owed him ten thousand talents, which was like saying he owed three trillion dollars. When Jesus was telling this story, the silver talent represented six thousand days' wages. So ten thousand of those would be close to sixty million days of wages today. That's a lot of punching the clock.[7] Jesus' hyperexaggeration is supposed to make us think it is a ridiculous amount of debt.

The king informed this guy that his wife, children, and possessions would be sold to pay off what he owed. This debtor fell to the ground, begging, "Pleeeease give me time. I wiiiilll pay you back!"

We know this guy would never be able to pay the king back. But the king was moved with compassion and forgave his entire debt! Like a country song backward, this guy got his wife back, his kids back, his house back, his dog back, his life back. The man didn't deserve it. The king just let him go.

And you wouldn't believe it, but this guy tracked down someone who owed him a few bucks. The contrast grabs ahold of you as this man who had been forgiven a massive amount grabbed hold of a guy's throat for owing him a five-spot. The huge-debt guy shouted, "Paaaay me back nowwww!" and the small-debt guy begged, "Pleeeease give me time, and I'llll pay you back!"

And what did huge-debt guy do? He threw small-debt guy in jail! So the forgiving king sent for him and said, "I canceled all that debt of yours because you begged me to. Shouldn't you have had mercy on your fellow servant just as I had on you?"[8]

Mercy should travel. It should be contagious. It should change a village. But that didn't happen. Instead, this guy hoarded mercy for himself with no intention of passing it on. So the king threw this ungrateful, unforgiving guy in the slammer. The debt that was once canceled was now back. This man had become his own torturer.

Maybe you understand what it is like to be your own torturer. I know I do.

The one person in my life I wanted to love me most I shut out because I could not forgive. The one person I wanted to be a part of my story, I wrote out of it. Like a will, like a death. But it would prove to be my own death, my own ill, my own fate. Everything inside of me wanted to let my father in, but instead, I saw the person I most wanted to choose me grow tired of trying. My unforgiveness imprisoned my peace, my joy, and my trust. And not just with my dad. I brought the sting of jail and my bitter heart into all of my relationships because that's what we do.

Lewis B. Smedes says, "To forgive is to set a prisoner free and discover that the prisoner was you."[9]

Our hearts become incarcerated by hate. Locked up by anger. Taken into custody by resentment. We think we are putting the one who hurt us in jail to suffer for what they did, but we aren't. *We* are the ones behind bars, and there's only one key that will get us out.

Letting go.

Friend, I understand you have been hurt. I understand you are mad as all get-out and have every right to be. I understand you can't get back what you lost. But this way of life, throwing them in jail, finds you sharing the cell!

If you are as bitter and angry and hurt as I was, if you are longing for love and pushing it away at the same time, if you are wanting those who hurt you to hurt too, there is only one direction you can turn to feel free. Let go of your need to be right, your need to go back and rewrite the story, your need to watch them sit in regret. And walk toward forgiveness.

Jesus knew that forgiving my father was what I needed in order to experience even more healing. Karolyn, my counselor, said I should write a letter to my dad. She said I didn't have to mail it but that it would help me get to a place of forgiveness. Ironically, my dad had an immense distaste for Christianity, and not only was I seeing a Christian counselor, but I made sure he knew it was his fault I needed counseling so he could foot the bill. The joke was on both of us because it was in these "rebellious" Christian counseling sessions that I began to hear about Jesus' call to forgive. God knew I wasn't looking to forgive my dad and my dad wasn't looking for God to forgive him. But God also knew that me forgiving my dad would release us both.

It took lots of rough drafts to write my truth. I had no intention of ever sending my "Where were you whens" and "Why weren't you heres." My hurt and blame and anger filled pages and pages.

I learned along the way, and a thousand times since, that putting voice to our pain is the only way to get to peace. My dad and I had to go *through* the pain, not around it. Jesus did that too. He had to go through the pain to get your peace and mine.

After Karolyn and I processed my letter, she encouraged me to send it, but for months I couldn't do it. What if he hurt me even more by denying his part in my pain? But one day, I took the risk. I folded up my heart, placed it in an envelope, and put it in the mail. Those words could only have been written with the help of a God who loved His enemies, prayed for those who persecuted Him, and forgave those who betrayed Him. I decided, regardless of how my dad chose to react, I would choose to be the kind of person I wanted to be. Our forgiveness can't be about the response of the person who hurt us. It has to be about our response to the God who heals us.

Peter started this conversation by asking, "How much pain do I have to go through before I can give up?" Let's pause and really think about Jesus. Let's think about all the people He came for, the people He collided with, the pain He would endure. Consider all the religious judgment, the expectations, the betrayal, the accusations, the mocking, the torture. I wonder if Jesus didn't ask the exact same question Peter did . . . "How much pain do I have to go through before I can give up?"

We will see that Jesus never does give up.

The story Jesus told Peter was a story about a king who lets go, told by a God who lets go. Jesus Himself would let go of being betrayed over and over again by this very same Peter.

This is a God who lets go of transgressions as far as the east is from the west. He lets go of our no-show selfishness, our damaging waywardness, our empty promises, and even our dark, dark bitterness. God does not hold a grudge. He is the God of a clean slate. He is in the habit of giving second, third, and one hundredth chances.

The over and over again of forgiveness can only come from a well that goes much deeper than your own. You can only draw it from the One who lets go of all of the ways we wound. When you run into His compassion, His grace, His love that forgives, you can't help but eventually do the same.

I saw my dad's handwriting on an envelope in my mailbox. He wrote me back. Terrified to open it, I sat down to handle whatever I might find. I tore the seal and pulled out his letter. There were words and words that strung together into the most humble, sad, sorry, regretful "I wish with everything I have that our story had written differently" letter. He owned that he hadn't been there for me like he should have been. He agonized over it. Absence broke his heart too. His "whys" were tied into his own pain and mess, failure and mistakes. He talked about how much he loved me and how hard it had been to not be there and how much he wished it could have been different. He said sorry and asked for my forgiveness, expressing a desire for relationship with me.

The most damaging misconception about forgiveness is that it's like trading in grief for an "it's all good." But forgiveness doesn't dismiss the pain you feel. Forgiveness doesn't make a father's absence OK. Forgiveness doesn't say you're making too big of a deal of it. No, forgiveness is letting go of the wounder. But grief, that's letting in the Healer. We don't grieve *or* forgive. We grieve *and* forgive.

I sat reading those words and just lost it. I had to grieve the blank pages of the past, and sometimes I still do. Forgiveness doesn't make them go away. But forgiveness is the only chance we have to write new pages. In that moment, I forgave my dad. I gave up a lifetime of resentment. My bitterness was swept away, and when it threatens to come back and arrest me, I turn to the One who prayed on that torturous cross, "Father, forgive them, for they know not what they do."[10]

This forgiveness thing was what gave our blank pages possibility. And the same is true for you. A new story is waiting for you once you finally set yourself free.

Forgiveness might not be instantaneous. It might not be easy. It might not even sound desirable, but walking toward forgiveness will set *you* free. How do I know? I know because Jesus told us so and showed us so. He made sure we knew that forgiveness is our direction, our way, our habit, our over and over again.

If you aren't there today, what is one step you can take to walk toward it?

When my friend was eleven, his dad committed suicide. I bet you can imagine what such a collision does to a little boy. Talk about blank pages. Your whole life, you wonder why you weren't enough for your dad to choose life. Derek spent his whole life thinking his dad would rather be dead than be his dad. He grew up with so much shame about it that he tried to keep this part of his story secret. In college, someone gave him a Bible. Derek heard the invitation Jesus lays out to forgive, and he thought, *I could never follow Jesus because I could never forgive my dad.*

For some crazy reason he felt led to sit on the steps of Old Main Hall on campus and strike up a conversation with a God he wasn't sure he believed in.

He said, *Hey God, can You get my dad on the line?*

Derek told his dad that he loved him and missed him and forgave him. He cried for the first time since his dad had passed, ten years before. He began experiencing God releasing him from the shame and unforgiveness he had felt his entire life. He saw the walls he had built to protect himself come crashing down. He began to receive love from people and from God, both of whom he had previously pushed away.

Forgiveness feels impossible, and yet Jesus calls us to live as though it is possible. We are called to forgiveness, not in an obligatory or fake way, but in a real, live, *Get the person who hurt me the most on the line, I need to let them off the hook* way. God calls us to forgive the people who hurt us because He knows *we* need it for *our own* healing.

Your first step might look like writing a letter you never send. It might look like setting foot into therapy. It might look like saying out loud, "I am angry." It might look like giving your own story permission to be told. It might look like taking an inventory of what you even need to forgive or telling the person who wounded you how badly you had been hurt. It might look like accepting the invitation to the family Thanksgiving you've been declining or sitting next to your ex at your kid's game and cheering for your child together. It might look like receiving someone else's "I'm sorry" by finally responding with an "I forgive you." It might look like coming back to the church and trusting healing is possible in a place you've been deeply wounded.

All I know is that waiting to wake up and "feel" forgiving on a random Tuesday is never going to happen. You might need to do an about-face toward the person who hurt you. And then take one step in the direction of forgiveness, and then another and another.

Jesus told the parable of the unforgiving debtor almost as if to say, "Let your life tell a different story than this one." Let your life look like our merciful King, who always lets go, never gives up, and forgives over and over again. Keep colliding with Jesus. Let His mercy cover every word that was never written. Allow His love to help you fill new pages. Take one small step in the direction of forgiveness. Jesus will meet you there and help you make room for a new story.

16

getting unstuck

On a rainy summer day, in an effort to keep my kids off street-sold Ritalin and for the sake of our sanity, I took them to the Fun Zone. It's this big warehouse full of bouncy houses, and kids run around, scream, sweat, and jump while the parents sip coffee and surf the web. When it was time to leave, I ran to the bathroom before gathering my kids. If you have children, you understand. Getting them out the door of someplace fun is as challenging as getting your great-grandma to do a marathon.

Facing the bouncy houses with a room full of parents watching their kids play, I hollered, "Aidan! Bella! It's time to goooo! Aidaaaan . . . Belllla . . ."

"One more time, Mommmm! Just one more time downnnn?"

I let them go *one* more time. Right then, I felt a tap on my shoulder, and I turned to see a Fun Zone employee. "Ma'am? Ummmm, maaaa'am, your skirt . . ." she said, repeatedly pointing at me. "Your skirt is stuck in your underwear."

She was right: My skirt was full-on tucked into my undypants—my way too old, holey, bottom-of-the-barrel, haven't-done-laundry undies—showing my cottage cheese thighs to a watching crowd.

This was my worst freaking nightmare.

Let me tell you, people. Sometimes in life we just need someone to tap us on the shoulder and let us know our skirt is stuck in our underwear. We all get stuck. We get stuck in rush hour traffic and stuck in dresses we can't get off. We get stuck with the check, with crazy roommates, and with bad hairstyles. We get stuck on blind dates with creepy people who drool and wanna make out. But when you and I find ourselves truly, truly "don't know how to get out of this" stuck, it can be paralyzing.

We can get stuck in commitments. We can get stuck playing the martyr, the people pleaser, or the overachiever. We can get stuck counting on something we shouldn't for pleasure, drinking wine to ease our stress, and telling white lies to cover our mistakes. We can get stuck in toxic friendships, and Lord knows, we can get stuck in family dysfunction.

I sit with people all the time who are stuck, but I'm not immune. I spent years stuck, trying to figure out how to love my mom outside that closet without letting her wounds bleed all over me. I was stuck in her denial, which led to countless run-ins, putting up with her drunken shenanigans.

I'd be whipping up lunch for the kids, and a simple phone call would totally trigger me. Mom would drunk dial, wanting a friend for the loneliness her drunkenness caused. Sometimes I avoided her. Then I would feel guilty. I would beat myself up about *What an awful daughter I am*, *What a poor example of Christ I am*, and *I probably caused her to drink because now she probably feels alone*. Other times, I would pick up the phone, and she'd be sweet and thoughtful, asking how the kids were and telling me about some delicious dish she just made. Her food was predictably amazing, but her behavior wasn't.

One vacation, Mom got plastered and then undressed in the living room in front of Rob and me. Of course he graciously shook it off to avoid shaming her, but I was over it. The next day, she got silly headbands out and had all of us wear them while we opened presents. The kids thought she was so fantastic that they named her "Crazygramcracker."

Mom would be in a terrible mood when she was sober because her body needed the drink. So, sober, I didn't like her, and drunk, I didn't either. I knew Jesus loved my mom, and I could find parts of me that loved her too. Some days I would try, and other days I wouldn't. We were as stuck as a mother and daughter could be.

Maybe you get it because you're stuck in your own ways too.

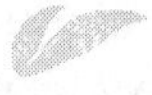

There's a guy in the Bible who gets us. He was stuck for nearly forty years.[1] And something changed when he collided with Jesus. But I want to start this story by telling you how it ends. Yep, I'm gonna be *that* guy. Jesus got this man unstuck, and that got Jesus very, very stuck. In fact, this collision catalyzed Christ's crucifixion.

John tells us, "That really set them off. The Jews were now not only out to expose him; they were out to *kill* him."[2] And in case you're thinking this caught Jesus by surprise—it didn't. Jesus showed up to a pool party on purpose, to heal this man.

This pool party wasn't exactly like the ones we picture. There were no beach balls, bikinis, and mai tais. There were sick people—blind, lame, and paralyzed. This place was called Bethesda, which means "house of mercy."[3] This pool promised a chance at healing. It was believed that an angel would stir the waters, and the first one to make it in afterward would be healed. So the broken and sick lined up like Bieber's Beliebers waiting for a backstage pass.

Most likely, Jewish religious leaders would have had real issues with this local superstition.[4] And I get that. It was a place that promised that the healthiest person is most likely to get well. What a limited offer of help! And look who was about to stir the waters with some drive-by healing.

There was a man at the pool who'd been an invalid for thirty-eight years. Stories of healing in ancient times often mentioned the years a person was sick to put an exclamation point on the *awesomeness* of the healer.[5] The Bible says Jesus "learned" of his condition, which could mean he was told by others. But beyond that, He sees into hearts and minds, and He clearly saw what we don't in this text. We begin to realize there was more going on with this guy than being physically sick. He was, in part, the cause of his own issues, and in fact, Jesus later warned him that if he continued to sin, life would get more difficult. Jesus clearly understood this man was his own hang-up.

And we can be our own hang-up too.

Jesus asked this man a piercing question: "Do you want to get well?"[6] This word *want* is the Greek word *thélō*, meaning not only "to will something," but also "to press on to action."[7] In other words, you do more than *want* to get well. You *move toward* getting well.

"Sir," the man replied, "I have no one to help me into the pool when the water is stirred. While I am trying to get in, someone else goes down ahead of me."[8] This guy was thinking about everything he couldn't do, rather than everything he could. He was comparing himself to others, and man, that landed him at a pity party. A friend of mine says, "You can show up to the pity party—but don't stay long." This guy might have camped out at that party for years. Instead of utilizing the help right in front of him, he chose to complain about people who had it better than he did. We do that too, don't we? We get stuck in negativity and blaming. We get stuck in learned helplessness, thinking, *I haven't had success, so I'll never have success. It never works out, so it will never work out. I always get hurt, so I will always get hurt.* We get stuck needing help and never asking.

This guy was so hyperfocused on *one thing*—the stirring water—that he missed *the* One Thing, the Healer standing right in front of him. Notice, this guy didn't actually answer Jesus' question. It sounds like he had given up believing that getting well was possible.

There are psychological studies that explain why we often get stuck. When we experience threat, danger, or pain, our brain has a built-in *fight*, *flight*, or *freeze* response. These are survival instincts. We fight the attacker, we run from the threat, or we freeze because we don't know what else to do. We get stuck because we experienced something traumatizing, and we get fastened there as though time stopped the moment we incurred the pain.[9]

When there is a risk of getting hurt again, we go into a mental place of survival without even knowing we are doing it. We stop trying to make friends because we're just going to move again. We create tension so people don't get close because getting close always hurts. We layer our body with more and more weight so no one will ever touch us that way again. We pick fights ever since we lost that one. We break up with a job every time a promotion is on the line so we don't risk not getting it.

The survival instinct that once protected us can begin to harm us. The thing we needed to survive *their* manipulation, *their* anger, *their* betrayal in the past can become the very thing that keeps us stuck in the present. These learned behaviors can overprotect, limit connection, erode our ability to trust, and cause countless other issues.

The thing about Jesus is that He sees how hurt we have been and how that pain is still wounding us, and He cares. So that's right where He shows up. Jesus said to the man at the pool, "Get up! Pick up your mat and walk."[10]

I can just hear this guy, "Uh . . . didn't You get the memo, Jesus? I don't move. I am the guy that sits here." Jesus doesn't see our stuckness the way we do. Jesus let this guy know what I think He wants to let us know:

You will have to move to get unstuck.

This man was probably no different than us. His survival brain might have been saying, *No, don't do it. Just stay here. Protect yourself from more hurt.* He would have had to move from being known as the guy who didn't move to the guy who did. What a risk! But boy, did it pay off!

The Bible describes this collision: "At once the man was cured; he picked up his mat and walked."[11] Jesus did in an instant what this guy had hoped for decades the stirring waters would do. Jesus healed his body, but don't forget this man still had to move from the place he had been camped out for years.

I met with this girl once who was in one of the saddest ruts you've ever seen. Her dad had died weeks prior, and I saw how paralyzed she was by this loss. She hadn't returned home to her husband and kids since her dad's passing. She had stopped going to work. Her grief had her incapacitated. The more layers of the story she peeled back, the more I understood why.

Her dad had been an alcoholic. He had been her whole life. She and her husband had often tried to help him out, and they had recently taken him in, in the hopes that he would get his act together. He called her one day from work and said he was thinking of going back to his place and wondered if she could look for his keys. Irritated, she said, "No! I won't look for your keys!"

I got her. You get to a point where you have been so, so hurt and you are so over covering, enabling, and caretaking. You get so sick of being the parent when you are supposed to be the kid, and you have these moments where you speak up, you protest, you let them know how you feel. And that's what she had done. She had chosen not to do for her dad what he could do for himself.

This woman said to me in the middle of a coffee shop, "I killed my dad!"

I was shocked. "What do you mean?"

Trying to hold it together, she told me more of the story. "That night he went out drinking and then, because he didn't have his keys, he walked up the back steps of his house and fell to his death."

"And you know what? I found his keys. The next day. They were right there. How could I not have looked for them? If I had given him his keys, he'd be . . ." She was stuck in grief, torture, and self-blame.

And here we sat, two strangers colliding, both wounded by the same sickness. All I wanted was for her to be embraced by the One who had begun to bring comfort and healing to my hurting heart, the One who had been pulling me out of ruts I'd been sitting in since I was a little girl.

I asked her, "Have you been trying to rescue your dad your whole life?"

"Yes." One hundred percent yes.

She loved him. She understood what drove him to drink. She had seen his gentle and caring side. All she had ever wanted was to be close to her dad. And yet he kept screwing up. And here she was, an adult, still trying to rescue, still trying to rely on him as the dad she had always needed. And now she was stuck in her own prison. Stuck in self-torture. Stuck believing she didn't deserve her family. Stuck in unwarranted guilt. Stuck calling herself his killer.

I prayed. I sensed God's Spirit wanting to get her unstuck, but I didn't realize God would unstick me while I helped unstick her. I asked this woman, "Can you believe by faith that God is sovereign over life and death—that He is the Giver of life and the One who determines when it shall end?"

"Yes," she said.

"Can you believe that God loved your dad despite his struggles and sickness?"

"Yes, I think so," she said.

"Can you believe that in God's desire to love and be close to us that He would do anything to rescue us, even to our very last breath?"

"Yes," she said.

"Can you believe then that it was God's job to rescue your dad and not yours?"

"Yes," she sighed.

"Can you relinquish that responsibility that should never have been yours?"

Tears. "Yes."

"Can you believe that God loves you and doesn't want you to carry the weight of this pain that will keep you stuck in all your relationships?"

Deep breath in and out. "Yes."

As I was asking these questions of her, God was asking them of me.

Yes.

Yes.

Yes.

Sigh.

I can.

Tears.

Deep breath, yes.

Jesus showed up at that coffee date and unstuck us both. Sometimes all it takes is a slight move, a reframing, a new belief, an insight. This sweet young woman was able to walk out of our time together no longer consumed by the impossible role of being her dad's rescuer and the terrifying guilt that she hadn't been a good one. Her move to get well, by bravely meeting with a stranger, not only helped her return to her husband, her children, her job, and her life, but it helped me too.

Friend, is Jesus tapping you on the shoulder and telling you that you're stuck? Are you stuck in an unhealthy relationship? In harmful habitual behavior? In limiting beliefs?

Jesus makes it clear we have to *move* to get well. We can't waste decades putting our hope in the move of a miracle without doing any moving ourselves. We have to *participate* in our own healing.

Sometimes God asks you to take the next step. Sometimes moving is as simple as doing the tiresome physical therapy exercises or calling a doctor. Sometimes it's taking agency over your own dreams and moving from talking about them to doing them. Sometimes it's meeting with the pastor and forgiving him. Sometimes it's coming out of the silence that's protecting someone else and hurting you. Sometimes it's setting a boundary. Sometimes it's looking for what God is doing when all you can see is what He isn't. Sometimes the move is showing up weeks on end to a therapist to locate where you're stuck and why.

But all the time, it's moving. And moving always feels like a risk. Your brain or your comfort or your fear might all be telling you,

Don't move! The little girl in you who had to hide in a closet might be saying, *Stay in there so you're safe!* The woman in you who has had her trust broken might be saying, *Don't trust anyone!* The child of an alcoholic in you might be screaming, *Don't upset them!* But these survival instincts aren't serving you anymore. In fact, they are hurting you. Jesus meets you here—here in the fear of getting hurt and here in the desire to get healing. He will say over and over again, "You have to move to get well."

After the chick who worked at the Fun Zone that was no longer fun got my attention, I started laughing like a crazy woman, because it was either that or cry. I could stand there and do nothing while half-mooning the moms and dads, or I could move lickety-split. As fast as I could, I turned around and gave my new friend a one-arm hug and probably held on waaaay too long. I used her body as a shield from the crowd as I unstuck my skirt.

Friend, when a lady in a Fun Zone shirt or your spouse or your therapist or your boss or Jesus Himself taps you on the shoulder to let you know you might be stuck, it's time to move.

17

the power of b

My daughter Bella was playing with a few girls at a park when they decided to do gymnastics competitions and deemed one girl the judge. This is not a mom brag, but Bella was the only girl in the group who was a gymnast and had been for years. Put that in your back pocket for context. Each girl did a "routine" and the judge, who happened to be eight years old, handed out scores. She went down the line saying happily, "You get a ten. You get a ten. You get a ten." And then she got to Bella and said with spite, "And youuuu, you get a zeeeerrrro."

I had no idea this hurtful run-in had taken place until Bella started bawling on the way home. I was ticked. Everything I could think to say was everything a mom shouldn't. I was like, "A zeeeerrrro? Not eeeeven a five?"

When we got home, I sat Bella down and asked, "After that hurtful experience, what would be easy to believe about yourself?" She said things like:

"I'm not good enough."

"I'm a zero."

"Other girls are better than me."

I was keenly aware that Bella could experience this wounded collision as an eight-year-old and carry the pain right into her adult life. What is true for Bella is also true for us. Hurtful experiences lie to us, and those lies stick. We carry them into every decade, every opportunity, every room, every relationship, and every collision. If we don't heal the hurt, the hurt keeps hurting. And if we don't replace the lies, they keep speaking. One wounded collision causes so many more.

Like Bella, I had a hurtful run-in with some girls, only it was a bunch of moms.

So I found myself in therapy again. Again? Again.

Erik looked like someone's grandpa. He began our session with a warmth that invited my pain out. I told him I had experienced a terrible friendship breakup, and it had happened in a group of mutual friends. And they were all still friends. Just not with me.

Erik wanted me to name the event that led to the collapse of this relationship. I said, "Oh that's easy. It was straight out of a high school movie set in the '80s, only we were all in our forties." It had started with a text thread my husband and I had been ghosted on, about dinner and a football game, only to go to said game and see this group of friends all hanging out, without us. And like, big deal, right? People forget to text back. And you can't be invited to everything. But it had felt like a straight shot of rejection, right into the veins.

And I reacted.

I didn't invite *them* to something.

That move was less about making them feel how I felt and more about feeling like they must not want to hang with me, so I went and hung out with other moms. It was less about revenge and more about insecurity. Maybe you relate? Maybe insecurity has gotten the best of you too. Maybe it has made you do things you can't take back, things that set off a chain of events you wish you could delete from the timeline.

These women reacted to my reaction. Then we were all reacting to one another's reactions. It was a back-and-forth of rejection, pride, and insecurities . . . topped with made-up stories, exclusivity, stonewalling, avoidance, and unrealistic expectations—all crashing into each other, colliding, wrecking a friendship I truly valued.

I tried to be a big girl and talk to my good friend in the group. I thought a heart-to-heart would help. I tried to take responsibility for my own big feelings that had gotten the best of me. But I also tried to be real about how hurt I felt. I wish I could say this conversation had led to the outcome I had hoped for, but I think I had already been voted off the island because of my public display of insecurity. For years, there were more misunderstandings, more hard conversations, more shame, and more tears. This wasn't a group I could avoid. We bumped into each other weekly, and when we did, I was alone and they were together. I didn't belong, and they were the cool kids club. I sat sidelined at the sporting events, and they sat teamed up. Their kids were in the car pool and mine was now left out. At every single run-in, I was reminded that I was not enough and too much. Have you ever felt like that? Like there's something about you that is intrinsically not enough and too much all at the same time? If so, we are in good company. Maybe we can sit next to each other on the bleachers.

As I shared this painful experience, the counselor saw something that had been there for way too long. I hesitated to travel that many miles back and visit such old pain. But I knew if I didn't, I would remain stuck in this new pain.

Erik took out a pen and paper and drew the letters *A* and *C*. The *A* stood for the *activating event* or *trigger*. The *C* was the *consequence*, a response or reaction to an activating event or trigger.

Then he drew a big fat *B* between them. The *B* stood for *belief*, specifically *self-belief*.

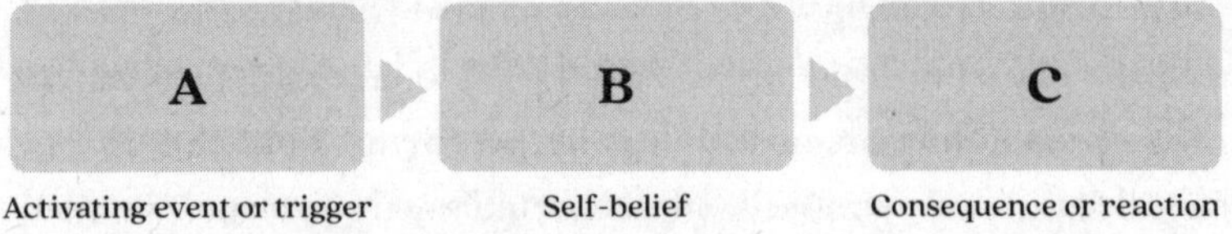

Erik used this *A-B-C* concept to illustrate the *power of belief*. He taught me that we don't get from *A* to *C* without *B*. We don't react to not getting an invite—by withdrawing or shutting down or some other wacky thing—unless we have a resident negative self-belief that's bossing us around and telling us what to do.

Erik suggested that I had reacted out of a wounded self-belief that had existed in me before I ever ran into the forty-year-old cool kids. And that wounded belief led to my wounded reactions, which triggered their wounded beliefs and reactions, which led to more wounded collisions, which had led to a mess. And look, I'm not tryin' to expose myself here because it's easy. This story is actually heart-wrenching. I lost one of my best friends, I cried about it forever, and I have to be real: A lot of it was because of me. Yes, some of it was because of them. It's embarrassing, and the only reason I am sharing it is because I have a feeling you might also be hurting the very people you want to love. Proverbs tells us just how powerful self-belief is: As she believes in her heart, so she is.[1] If you think you won't be chosen, you won't be. If you think you're average, you will be. If you think you aren't worthy of more, you won't be seen as worthy of more. If you believe you're inadequate, you will find all sorts of reasons to rule yourself out. If you believe you aren't cool enough, you might act all sorts of wonky out of insecurity, and then people will never see the true cool that *is* in you.

Self-belief might very well be our worst enemy, and yet it has the power to be our best friend—our *new* best friend.

I learned from Erik that we cannot control what events or collisions come our way, but we can change our reaction by changing our *belief.* Here's what this means: You can't change what you don't get invited to, but when you believe you're worthy of an invitation, you can change your reaction to being left out. You can't change your in-laws' continual passive-aggressive jabs, but when you believe you are "wonderfully made,"[2] you can change how you respond to criticism. You can't change a toxic coworker's attempts to polarize you, but when you believe your contribution matters, you can change your response to their drama.

My friend and I had collided. She had hurt me, and I imagined I also had hurt her. All I was sure of was that I needed God to heal my *B*. Maybe you need God to heal your *B* too?

At one point in my processing with Erik, it was like I stepped on a land mine. I told him, "This whole thing takes me back to when I was fifteen."

Erik asked, "What were you doing when you were fifteen?"

I told him the whole story. When I had moved to my aunt and uncle's house, leaving my mom, my friends, my house, my room, my school, my pets, my sports teams, my everything, I had walked into a new high school and sat in the bathroom stall at lunch. I wanted to hide that I was alone so no one could make me feel I deserved to be, more than I already did.

The cool girls all sat together at the same table. I would have done anything to be invited to sit at *any* table. I ventured into the lunchroom one day to grab something to eat. I was sporting my black-and-cream-striped sweater, feeling like I had one of my best 'fits on for sure. And out of nowhere, an apple whacked me in the head. Some dingus from the popular table thought it might up his stock to tag me right 'side the noggin. A laughing lunchroom with nowhere to sit, no people to speak up, no one to walk beside—that hurt like nobody's business. And it *was* nobody's business. No one knew who I was, what I was going through, where I came from, or how awfully triggering this apple incident was.

Trying not to bust out in public tears, I skipped food and walked out, acting like I could care less. I headed to my bathroom stall, trying not to come apart. I wanted to call my mom. I wanted to go back to my friends, my house, my room, my school, my pets, my sports teams, my name. I would have gone back, even to the hard, because at least it was a hard I had known.

Erik asked, "How did that make you feel, to be given up on by your mom?"

"It made me feel like it's easy to give me up for something else, like I'm disposable and unwanted, like I'm clearly not worth keeping . . . Exactly like this forty-year-old cool kids club makes me feel. Like . . ."

"I'm not good enough."

"I'm a zero."

"Other girls are better than me."

And there you have it, folks. This is why we pay counselors the big bucks. Erik helped me to see something that had been there all along:

a nasty belief that resides on the walls of my heart like the wallpaper you can't peel off the living rooms of turn-of-the-century homes.

I know I'm not alone in this. I know you probably believe some nasty lies about yourself too. We've all had wounded collisions that wounded our self-belief, and now our self-belief is wreaking havoc on our lives, causing more wounded collisions. So what do we do? Because let's be real . . . Our pep talks in the mirror, our rah-rah daily affirmations, our motivational memes on IG, and all the other ways we try to con ourselves into liking who we are, aren't doing the trick.

This is an age-old human condition.

In Matthew 8, a man who felt incredibly unworthy had a life-changing collision with the only One who can heal our wounded beliefs.[3] Jesus entered Capernaum, and this man, a centurion, ran to Him. This guy served in the Roman army and was most likely in charge of a hundred soldiers. As a leader he would have had great respect. But outside of work, he would have been seen as an oppressor by the Jews.

Gentiles like this centurion were seen as dirty, despicable, and irreligious. Some religious Jews would pray each morning, "I give thanks that I am a man and not a woman, a Jew and not a Gentile, a free man and not a slave."[4] The devout would not have hung at this guy's house, as it was considered unclean. They wouldn't eat his tacos or drink his margaritas. Imagine what he probably believed about himself. His collisions could have left him feeling like he, too, was not enough, too much, and didn't belong.

The centurion had every reason to assume that Jesus wouldn't do him any favors. The centurion's negative self-belief could have kept him home, but he chose to come to Jesus anyway, to get help for someone he cared about.

He got right up in Jesus' grill and said, "Lord. My servant is at home, paralyzed and in terrible pain." This word *Lord* comes from the word *kurios*, meaning "he to whom a person belongs."[5] This dirty, despicable centurion who likely had only heard he *doesn't* belong said to Jesus, "I belong to You."

You know, it's a pretty vulnerable thing to belong to someone. To belong to a spouse or a friend group or a church . . . or a Lord . . . is wholly vulnerable and risks complete rejection. And yet isn't belonging what we all want? Did Jesus clap back with a "You're not invited"? Did He say, "You can't sit with us" or "You're not good enough to be My kinda people"? No! Jesus offered to go with him.

You can see the power of *B* at play here because even when Jesus offered to enter his life, the man said, "Lord, I do not deserve to have you come under my roof."[6] Some of us have been told over and over again how unworthy and unwanted we are, so much so that we could be standing in the presence of God Himself, and He could be offering to come into our lives, and we would still RSVP: undeserving. But Jesus just won't have it. When Jesus collided with the centurion, He did business with this man's wounded beliefs. His presence, His willingness, and His words spoke truth over this man like:

"You are worthy."

"You're invited."

"You belong to Me."

"And, yes, I belong to you."

The centurion said to Jesus, "Just say the word, and my servant will be healed. For I myself am a man under authority, with soldiers under me. I tell this one, 'Go,' and he goes; and that one, 'Come,' and he comes."[7]

Jesus heard this, and the Bible says He was amazed. This was a man who had been made to believe he wasn't enough to come into the presence of God, into the places of worship of God, into relationships with people deemed godly, yet he boldly believed that God could just say a word and heal his friend. Jesus said in front of a watching crowd who looked down on this man, "I have not found anyone in Israel with such great faith."[8] Then Jesus slapped one more truth on this man:

"You are astonishing."

Jesus knew that this man had a wounded self-belief, but what astonished Him was that this man came anyway. The lies he believed about himself didn't hold him back like they so often hold us back. Our wounded self-beliefs get in our way—they hinder and harm us, and they even hinder and harm the good we can do in the world. This man believed in Jesus and what Jesus could do more than he believed in his own inadequacy.

And that was what astonished Jesus.

Jesus said to the centurion, "Go! It will be done just as you believed it would." And the Bible says the servant was healed that hour. Talk about the power of belief! Because this man ran to Jesus despite his feelings of unworthiness, not only was his power of belief healed, but he was also used to help heal someone else.

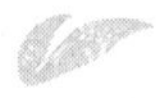

The day Bella was told she was a zero, we went home and wrote down on Post-it notes every possible negative thing she *could* believe from her wounded collision on the playground.

"I'm not good enough."

"I'm a zero."

"Other girls are better than me."

We named each lie, and there she was, covered with the stuff.

Then I unstuck every single one and replaced them with truths. I proclaimed who God says she is all over her:

"You are God's daughter."

"You are fearfully and wonderfully made."

"You are God's workmanship."

"You are a child of God."

"You are God's beloved."

The next thing you know, Bella was standing there blanketed in beautiful truths.

Maybe you are covered in wounded self-belief Post-it notes too.

Jesus is in the business of healing beliefs—the ones that hurt and still hurt, the ones you picked up on the playground decades ago and the ones you picked up last week. At every collision, He unsticks the stinging lies and replaces them with the absolute truth from heaven that you are worthy. And when we allow Jesus to heal our *B*, we can heal our daughters' *B*'s so they become women who react to all their collisions from a place of belonging rather than a place of rejection.

So friend, I want to invite you, like I did Bella, to be a child of God who believes the truth. It starts with recognizing the lies you've picked up along the way. You can't just slap truths on them. We do that, you know? We try to hype ourselves up with pep talks, but that doesn't take away the lies. The harder work is to locate your wounded beliefs, the ones you unknowingly picked up and are living out of, the ones that are taking a wrecking ball to your life. You have to name them and take them off. Then you can splatter yourself with truths.

This is not a onetime thing. We need to run to Jesus every time we feel unworthy. If you have to do it every day, do it every day. If you have to do it every five minutes, do it every five minutes. If you have to do it just when you run into the cool kids club, do it. Run to

Jesus. Bring Him all the ways you believe you aren't enough, all the ways you've been told you're too much, all the reasons you have never belonged. Stand in His presence and let Jesus dismantle every one of the false narratives you have believed about yourself. Allow Him to declare over you worth upon worth upon worth. Watch while He replaces every last nasty lie with beautiful truths, till you're covered head to toe.

Let Jesus heal your wounded self-belief—and then be astonished by the power your *B* has to help heal others.

18

get out of the boat

I was speaking at a church about brokenness, and an older man with glasses wanted to talk afterward. He said that one day, his wife had locked herself in her sewing room. When I picture women with sewing rooms, they make quilts and drink tea and talk about their grandchildren. But his wife wouldn't come out. At first he checked on her calmly, but he got worried when she failed to answer, so he finally broke the door down. There he had found his bride with blood pouring out of her wrists. No one else in his giant church knew because somehow when we share this kind of story, it distances us from people.

Years ago, I led a group of college students on a service trip to a street church in Vancouver, British Columbia. One night we were tasked with serving hot dogs and leading chapel. Men and women who were high, crazy, stinky, dirty, and angry showed up to get some food in their systems before they headed back out to the war zone they called home. I will never forget my excitement to change the world, one hot dog at a time. There I was, the smiling hot dog honcho, when a big, tough guy with long, greasy hair and bloody sores started yelling at me, "Why is your God still on the cross with blood all over Him? I thouuuught He rohhhhse from the deeeead?" He was referring to a horrific icon, hanging above the hot dogs, of a bloody Christ on the cross, wondering why my God was absent from his pain.

I showed up to speak at a summer camp and was immediately warned about the young man who had just gotten out of a psych ward he'd been admitted to for trying to kill himself. One morning, after I had finished speaking, I was walking the trail back to my cabin when I noticed this kid walking behind me. I slowed down and asked how he was doing. He started getting really angry. He paced around me, clenching his fists, putting words to his pain: "Why do I have to have my dad? He beat my mom. I swear I will kill him. He's in prison and when he gets out . . . You don't know how hard it is to be a Black man. You don't know the things I go through, Willow."

He punched the tin roof of an outbuilding. I stood present, listening but truly scared. With a bleeding hand, he said, "I want to die. My brother is dead. I just want to go be with him. I think about killing myself."

Entering people's pain is intimidating, scary, and hard. It can be triggering, and it can make you feel like you have little to offer people with serious struggles. And yet that's exactly who Jesus goes chasing down on purpose. In Mark 5, Jesus went out of His way to collide with a man whose pain would be incredibly overwhelming for most of us.[1] Jesus got out of a boat and visited a cemetery, which was taboo for a Jewish person. Tombs were considered unclean, but that didn't stop Jesus from walking into this home sweet home for troubled outcasts.[2]

As soon as Jesus set foot on shore, a naked homeless man ran toward Him and fell at His feet. The Bible says this man had been "chained hand and foot, but he tore the chains apart. . . . No one was strong enough to subdue him. Night and day among the tombs and in the hills he would cry out and cut himself with stones."[3]

This word *subdue* comes from the word *damazō*, which means "to tame a wild animal."[4] People were trying to tame this man like a beast, probably for the same reasons *we* bind and chain people. They scare us and make us uncomfortable. When people are hurting and then isolated, they begin to self-harm, sabotage, numb, hide, create chaos, and cry louder. This downward spiral leads to more isolation, pain, and sickness.

THE DOWNWARD SPIRAL OF PAIN

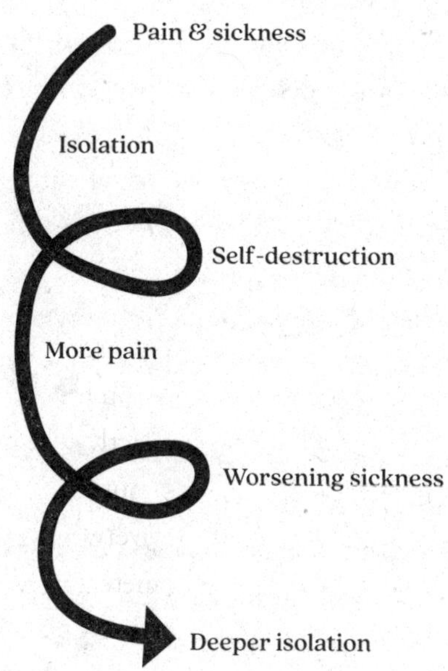

As soon as this guy in a spiral saw Jesus walk into his hood, he came running toward Him, shouting, "What do you want with me, Jesus, Son of the Most High God?"[5] The words "Most High God" were used in the Old Testament to call out the supremacy of the one true God over all the counterfeit, do-it-yourself, pretend gods.[6] So often, Jesus had to answer questions and make statements to get people to understand who He was but not with this guy. This guy, in his deranged, desperate state, knew exactly who Jesus was and what Jesus could do. And he begged Jesus not to take His power out on him.

This man had been tortured by demons and tortured by people ostracizing him. He must have wondered, *Will Jesus be any different from His people?* I think this is a question a lot of people ask when they have been pushed out and left for dead. That's what we do—we project our experiences with other people onto God. But God is not the pastor who used you. He is not the ex-boyfriend who cheated on you. God is not your dad who controlled you, and He's not the church that shamed you. A wounded view of God has us expecting Jesus to be just like the people who hurt us. But look at who Jesus really is. He runs directly into the tombs where we're cut off and in pain. He cares that we are spiraling, and He wants to restore our broken view of Him, ourselves, and the people who hurt us.

Here, we see that Jesus went out of His way to collide with a cutter who viewed God as a torturer. And you know what the first thing Jesus said to this guy was?

"What is your name?"

Jesus didn't treat him like a wild animal. He didn't whip out the divine handcuffs and lock him up. Jesus acknowledged this man's worth. He had an identity, a story, a heart. He was a creation of God. Someone's child. Someone's brother. He mattered. Even his name mattered.

The man answered, "My name is Legion . . . for we are many."[7]

"Legion" is a Latin word for a Roman army unit of about six thousand soldiers. The Romans had been oppressing the Jewish people. This man's very name suggested his severe oppression. It's almost as though he was identifying with feeling tormented.[8] It was like he said, "My name is An Army Dominates Me." It reminds me of the people you and I are scared to collide with. It's like they tell us, "My name is No One Can Know." "My name is I Did Something I Can Never Undo." "My name is I Might Kill Myself."

Shockingly, Legion was begging Jesus not to send his demons away. He knew Jesus had the power to take away the very thing that made him feel crazy, but like many of us, this man was more comfortable with the oppression he was used to than the freedom he wasn't. But Jesus wants freedom for us.

When Jesus persisted in healing the man, the demons asked to be sent into some pigs hanging out nearby, and Jesus gave them what they asked for. You would think watching those oinkers rush off a cliff and drown in the sea would be cause for celebration. But the pig farmers most likely saw all the lost profit from the Christmas hams they could have sold, and they ran into town reporting what had happened. They were probably pretty ticked off about what Jesus had just done to their economy. The entire community came running back like paparazzi, and guess what they saw? This man they once saw as a madman was sitting there, dressed, "in his right mind."[9]

And they weren't happy about it.

This miracle scared people! So the townspeople begged Jesus to leave their region. They feared the power of evil, but even more, it appears they feared the power of God! Look at what fear did throughout this story. It does the same thing in *our* lives. Fear identifies us by our pain and sickness. Fear pushes us into isolation. Fear keeps us oppressed.

And fear keeps God at a distance.

As Jesus got into the boat to leave, this man begged to go with Him. This is one of the coolest moments in any collision I have ever seen. A man whose life had been wrecked by darkness. A grave dweller, scarred and cut, crying out, left to live alone with the dead, outside of all relationship. A man who had once begged for his demons, now begged for Jesus.

To our surprise, this Jesus who calls us to follow Him did not let this man hop in the boat. Instead, Jesus encouraged him to turn the lights back on. To enter, as brave as it sounds, back into community. To boldly testify about Jesus' healing to the very people who had broken him. Wow, none of us wants to return to the people and places that hurt us! But following Jesus doesn't always look the way we expect, and neither does healing. Jesus shows us: Further healing banks on moving from isolation back into relationship.

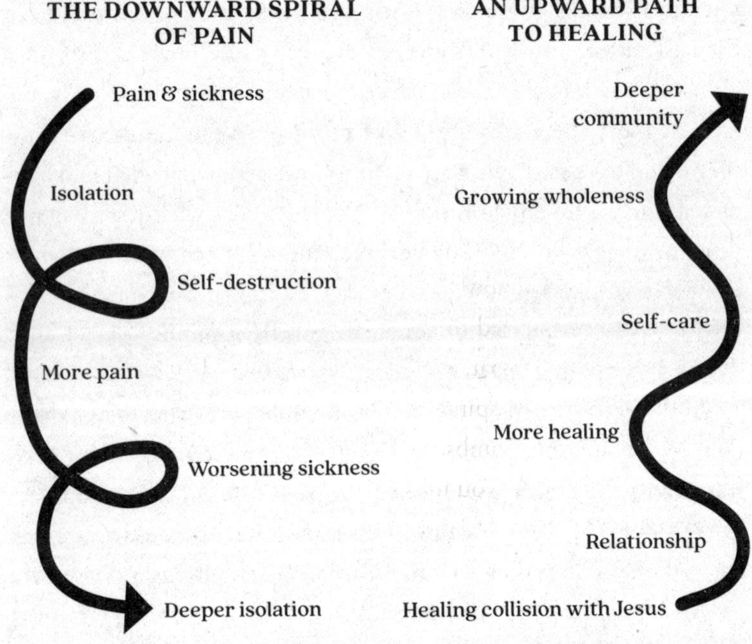

This man who had once been in a vicious cycle with no apparent off-ramp went into the Decapolis, the ten nearby cities, and the masses were amazed. Jesus interrupts the spiral. He disturbs graveyards. He redirects trajectories. He enters a person's downward path of pain and sets into motion an upward path to healing that might bring healing for others too.

Notice Jesus called Himself "Lord." He is not a mere magician, an exorcist, or a Jewish teacher. Jesus was saying, "I am God and a God of mercy." Contrary to what our wounded collisions with people who claim to be Christians have shown us, Jesus is merciful. He is a God who cares. A God who enters pain. A God who wants to free you, not chain you. A God who won't tame you like an animal but wants to know your name. And He is a God who calls *you* to be merciful, as He is, in all your collisions with wounded, wounding people.

So let me turn the heat up in here: Where were Jesus' followers in this story?

They were still in the boat.

Right before Jesus healed this cutter, He rescued His disciples from a terrible storm.[10] You know the one—the disciples were crying like wee babies, and Jesus showed the wind and waves who's boss. Right after that, they docked the boat, and Jesus stepped out to collide on purpose with this man who was spiraling. But His followers didn't follow Him. Jesus walked into the tombs, and His followers stayed in the boat.

Look, you can't say you follow Jesus and not follow Jesus into the places He goes.

Following Jesus necessitates entering the pain, sadness, isolation, tombs, and cutting of others. So I have to ask you: Are you on the seashore waiting for Him to heal others while you protect yourself? Do you watch Jesus step into hard, dark places and hesitate to follow because you'd rather hang back with your friends, cozy where you are?

What will our running away from pain do to heal it? What will it do for the man whose wife is cutting herself in her sewing room? Nothing.

She still bleeds.

After we were done serving hot dogs, I saw the man who had yelled at me sitting alone at the chapel service. I was more than scared to sit next to him, but what was I doing volunteering at a street church if I was unwilling to sit next to street people? I sat down and watched our students lead worship. I started singing, and a few minutes later, I looked over and the angry man was weeping. Shaking, I put my hand on his back and patted it. In a tone that seemed too tender to come out of this massive man, he said, "You have a beautiful voice." Heroin does a lot of terrible things, but I never knew it makes you hard of hearing.

He said, "I miss my kids."

Well aware of what it's like to miss family, I said, "What is it going to take to get you home?"

This time he looked at me when he spoke. "I'm punishing myself—I deserve this."

Then he told me why he thought he warranted this torture. One night in a rage, he had purposely driven his truck into his house with his wife and kids *inside*. He had served time in prison and then left for the hills because men like this don't get invited over for supper.

This was a man who was now in the tombs punishing himself with no end to the misery. I wonder what that bloody Jesus on the cross might say about this man's pain? Must he suffer for his sins forever? All I know is that Jesus said, "This is my body, broken for you."[11]

After the kid from camp punched the tin roof, his knuckles began to bleed. He fell to his knees, hunched over, and started to cry. Of course I was scared, and of course I wished I could bounce and someone more qualified could step in. But what would running from pain do to heal it? All I had was the way of Jesus. I knew what He is like: He enters pain. So I stood with this kid for however long it took. I stayed there so he knew he mattered. So he knew he wasn't alone. So he knew God was with him.

We can't tell people God is with them if we are unwilling to be.

That week, the camp wrapped their arms around this kid, and it was a beautiful thing to behold. This kid who had just been in the psych ward was changing before our very eyes. Slowly, a smile sneaked out. He started opening himself up to hugs. And next thing you know, I saw him *giving* hugs! I watched him sing camp songs with all his might. And dance. I saw him dance. The last day, he came up to thank me. We had become buds. We hugged, and I held on. I wanted to give him something to take with him.

"Choose life.

God gave it to you.

You are meant to be here.

Don't forget it."

I hated having to say goodbye. He was headed back to the pain he came from, and guess what? He is gonna need some of God's people to step out of their comfort zones and set foot into his pain to keep reminding him to live. And the same is true for the husband and wife who can't share their story in church and the man wandering the streets torturing himself somewhere in Vancouver, British Columbia. Who will step out of their safe circle and enter the hills, the war zones, and the pews to make sure people know their names matter, their stories matter, their lives matter?

The guy in the tombs experienced a complete life change because Jesus set foot into a place others avoided. Friend, when you and I said yes to following Jesus, we said yes to getting uncomfortable, yes to entering darkness, and yes to hugging angry kids. We said yes to loving people who are hard to love and yes to serving as many hot dogs as it takes for even one person to know their life matters.

I wonder what would happen if, collectively, Jesus' people started following Him into the places and spaces He goes. Maybe our lives would tell more stories like this one.

There are people crying out.

Get out of the boat.

19

the ultimate wounded collision

Every single time Jesus collided with a wounded person and they were made more whole, an exchange took place. Jesus knew He would be hurt so they could be healed. I read once that Jesus worked miracles at His own expense. Not only did He bear "the ultimate cause of sickness, the sin of the world," but each healing "meant for him a fresh realization of what bearing" that meant.[1] It is staggering to think that Jesus knew at every collision when He healed someone that He would ultimately feel their pain. Who would do that? Who would intentionally keep healing people if it meant taking on their wounds?

When Jesus healed the man by the pool, He knew He would get stuck so this man could get unstuck. Jesus would be stuck by all the things that stick us: our pessimism, our pride, our fear, our patterns. He was willing to get in a rut so the man who hadn't moved in a lifetime could finally get out of one.

He would be arrested so we could go free.

When Jesus stood with the woman caught in adultery, He knew that ultimately it would be Him who would be condemned. He knew He would take on the blunt trauma of every stone He helped her escape. He would be punished for every walk of shame, every way we've felt naked, paid penance, stood guilty, stolen from others, stacked regrets, and sought to be wanted in unwanted ways.

He would be crushed by all our sin so we would know all our worth.

Jesus knew when Peter asked Him about forgiveness that He would have to forgive this disciple over and over. Jesus knew He would be betrayed by so many who claimed to follow Him—by the crowds that loved His miracles, by Judas for a measly thirty coins, by you, and by me. Still, this Lord took the blame. Stabbed in the back, sold out, left to hang by all the Peters, everywhere.

He would be faulted so we could be forgiven.

Jesus knew when He set foot in the tombs to show love to the man who was isolated and cutting himself that He would incur those wounds. Every way we feel we deserve the pain, the punishment, the consequence, Jesus endured. Every single cut we have made razed across His arms, His face, His back. Every moment we have ever self-debased, self-sabotaged, self-destructed—our bulimia, bankruptcy, addiction, masochism, withdrawal, overworking—all of it was on Jesus. All the ways we carve guilt, with or without a blade, slashed Him. Our self-inflicted gashes would be stitched up, and Jesus would bleed every last one for us.

He would be mercilessly whipped so we could end our self-harm.

When Jesus went to the party with the drunkards, gluttons, and swingers, He knew He would take on the judgment that spewed hate in that room. Every racist, discriminatory, slanderous, faultfinding criticism ever uttered pierced Jesus. Everything that has canceled anyone, every legalistic religious rant, every ugly word you've ever said about your neighbor flew at Jesus, nailing Him to a cross.

He would be hammered by our hate so we could be struck by His love.

When Jesus stopped for the man on the mat, the one whose friends lowered him through the roof, He knew He would take on that man's crippling paralysis and the things that hold *us* back. Every reason we were ever unable to move came on Jesus. Crowned, identified, named by our inabilities. Our jagged thorns, anxiety, depression, phobias, envy, insecurities—Jesus took on all of it. Jesus didn't have to help that man, but He did, knowing a transaction was in progress.

He would be powerless so we could be healed.

Jesus knew when He told the parable of welcoming home the lost son that He would be forsaken by the Father. Jesus knew the pig slop would be smeared all over Him. Every wayward, selfish, sloppy mile we've traveled away from the Father, Jesus made up by carrying that cross on His back to Calvary. His march toward suffering made sure we know nothing can separate us from the love of God.

He would be distanced so we could come home.

When Jesus went out of His way for the woman at the well, He knew quenching her thirst would parch Him. All the reasons we hustle, long, lust, crave, and sip dehydrated Jesus. He would cry on the cross, "I thirst," and they would soak a sponge in sour wine and lift it to Him on a hyssop branch.[2]

He would become thirsty so we would never have to draw from a nasty well again.

Jesus knew when He cured the centurion's servant that He would be struck by human frailty. Jesus would take on our weakness, contagion, vulnerability, and mortality. Our Immanuel—*God with us*[3]—would be manhandled, handcuffed, arrested, mocked, stripped, and would have to hand over His wants, His power, His life. Jesus would breathe His last breath and surrender, "Father, into your hands I commit my spirit."[4]

He would become like us so we would know He's with us.

Jesus wept with Martha and Mary. He knew what trading their sorrow would cost. When Jesus raised Lazarus back to life, He knew that He would take on Lazarus's death.

His life for our life, as Isaiah prophesied:

> Surely he took up our pain
>   and bore our suffering,
> yet we considered him punished by God,
>   stricken by him, and afflicted.
> But he was pierced for our transgressions,
>   he was crushed for our iniquities;
> the punishment that brought us peace was on him,
>   and *by his wounds we are healed.*
>
> ISAIAH 53:4-5, EMPHASIS ADDED

I often picture all of us He has collided with gathered at the foot of the cross. We've all heard the news, and we've followed Him here. The woman from the well is here, right alongside Mary and the centurion. I see the lepers and the woman caught in adultery, the man on the mat, and you, and me. Many are gathered—young and old, men and women, orthodox and irreligious, curious and hungry, doubtful and heartbroken, put together and poor, haters and lovers, people from every nation, every tongue, every tribe. I look around, and I see the woman who is afraid of heaven, and I see my old friend, the one I don't talk to anymore.

And the most unbelievable thing happens . . . I see the two thieves. They robbed the sense of safety right out from under their neighbors, and here they are, crucified alongside Jesus, who is offering them paradise. And I look over and see John, the man from my childhood who stole my safety, here at the cross. The anger that dragged my mom up and down the stairs, branding her naked body, brands Jesus. Every reason that man wanted to break Mom and me breaks Jesus on the cross. I see Him mocked by the mean boy in the alley, by all the meanies who have mocked any of us, by all the ways we've hurled insults at others.

I scan the faces, and I stumble in shock. From the cross, Jesus sees His mom. I see my mom too.

She's looking up at Jesus' absolute agony, and I see a moment where she comprehends that her own pain and everything that caused it is on Him. Whoever caused my grandmother Kathryn's pain that made her drown her sorrow in happy hour—those wounds are on the cross. The pain she inflicted on my dear mother is on Jesus. I see the bloody pain my mom caused me, and the pain I've caused others. And Jesus is willingly enduring it. And then I look over and see you comprehend that the person who wounded you the most—they are here. And the pain that causes their pain that caused yours is tormenting Jesus too.

He groans, "Father, forgive them, for they know not what they do."[5]

The abuse that made that woman with cancer afraid of God, even that is stripping Jesus. The woman who blamed herself for her dad's death—that blame is put on Christ, taken off her. He feels the grief of the woman who gave up her baby in secret. Jesus knows what it's like to be pierced, to undergo the sharp, unending pain my friend Derek knew, the stinging emptiness left by suicide laid bare on the cross. The mom on meth who was hurting her kids with what hurt her—all that hurt, woven into a crown of thorns, is placed on Jesus' head. The sins of the generations passed down from her parents to her, from ours to us, strike Jesus, damning Him to death. The sin that separated me from my father, all the sin that separates any of us from the love we were meant to have, Jesus feels it.

Jesus cries out, "My God, my God, why have you forsaken me?"[6]

On that cross is every reason people didn't show up for us. All the reasons they left us out. The ways they told us we deserved pain. On that cross is every reason we've ever believed the lie that we are unlovable and made others feel the same.

We are all watching Jesus wear the wounds that wounded us, that wound others.

And I realize that something Cindy used to tell me is true: "At the foot of the cross, the ground is level." I need the same thing my grandmother and my mother needed, the same thing we all need. We need the same thing that the person who hurt us needs. We all need a love that heals.

Here we are, side by side, witnessing the brokenness of humanity wiped all over Jesus. And we remember that He gave blind men sight, sent demons packing, stopped bleeding, and bossed storms around. We know He has power. He can tell this tsunami to end. He can speak a word, and it will be done. So why doesn't He save Himself when He saved so many others?

Jesus stays in the brokenness that drags Him up and down the stairs, naked and rug burned. He stays and lets His wrists bleed like those of the bride locked in her sewing room. He stays and is called every name you've ever been called. And you're here, at the foot of the cross, watching sweet Jesus go through all this. He chooses this suffering to say this to you:

"In case you didn't know, in case life has told you otherwise, I will do anything for you. I will give up My life so you can find yours.

I will take on your wounds. They will be on Me—they were never supposed to be on you. I won't run from your pain. I will run into every hurt that hurt you that hurt others."

"I will be broken so you can be made whole.

I'll be abandoned so you can be adopted.

I'll bear the accusations so you have an Advocate.

I'll endure insults so you can be held in approval.

I'll wear your shame so you don't have to.

I'll take the torture so you'll stop torturing yourself.

I'll be wrecked so you can be redeemed.

I'll shoulder the separation so we will always be close.

I'll give you everything I have so you know you're all I want."

Jesus wears our wounds. He doesn't run from our brokenness. He wipes it all over Himself. God runs into every wound that hurt you that hurts others, taking it upon Himself so you can walk away whole rather than broken.

You see Him, and you hear Him.

I do too.

And I wonder, *Can we let it sink deep into our souls?*

I look over at you.

I am so, so glad you're with me.

I reach over and whisper so you never forget: This is Love. This is the only Love that can truly heal what wounds us all. This is what you've been longing for. It is the *ultimate* wounded collision—the only painful run-in we will ever have that leaves us more whole than broken.

part 3

running toward pain to bring healing

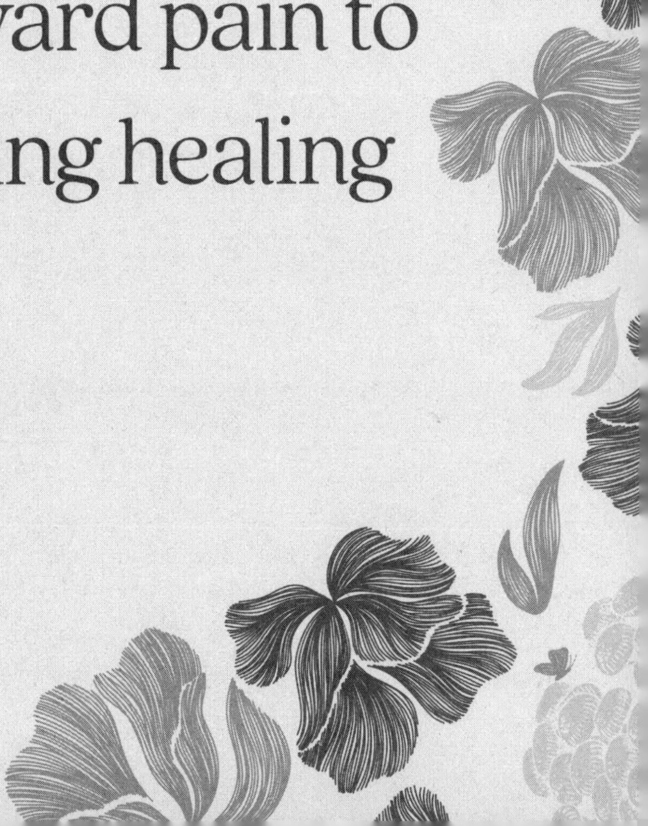

20

get off the bus

The more we collide with Jesus, the more we heal, and the more we heal, the more we become like Jesus. And the more we become like Jesus, the less we run *from* broken, messy, sinful, dysfunctional, toxic, hurting people and instead run *toward* them. We find ourselves chasing after people because all we want is for them to experience what we have: Jesus' rescue, help, hope, forgiveness, love, healing, and purpose.

When I worked in college ministry, I took teams of students on service trips during spring break. And I'll tell you this: There's nothing more life-changing and Jesus-adventuring than a week serving the poor and powerless. One year I got to serve with Sabby. She was one of the sweetest students I ever took on a trip. She was new in her faith, and it was so fun to see her eyes wide open to how Jesus would purpose her to help others.

The week after our trip, Sabby was doing her recycling job on campus. On her route, she found herself next to a dorm when a young man's body fell onto the concrete right in front of her.

This student had lost all hope and jumped out of the seven-story building, and Sabby was the first responder. He was still alive. She called 911, but when the medics got there, they pushed Sabby back, and she saw him take his last breath. For months, Sabby replayed the horror, the images and sounds, wishing she could go back and erase the whole thing, wishing she could have done more to save his life.

A few weeks later, Sabby was on a bus. Out the window, she saw a guy crying. The next time the bus stopped, she looked out and saw him again! She said to a girl she didn't know, "If we see that guy again, we should get off the bus and help him." I imagine that girl looked at Sabby like she was bonkers. But Sabby kept seeing the same man and knew God was telling her to do something. She got off the bus and went up and tapped him on the shoulder.

"What do you want?!" he said, agitated.

"Do you need anything?" she asked.

"Whaaaat do you wannnnt from me?" he said.

"I just want to make sure you're OK. Do you want to talk?"

Sabby sat on the curb of some sidewalk with a man she'd never met while he poured out his life story. Two hours later, he said to her, "I was on my way to kill myself before you came after me. Why did you?"

Stunned that she was encountering another suicidal man, she said, "I believe Jesus takes care of people when they are hurting, and He sent me."

Rob and I went on a two-week honeymoon to Mexico. After a week of lounging by the pool and drinking piña coladas, we got bored. Not with each other but with living for ourselves. Don't get me wrong, I do love a good week of vacay. But we were itchin' for something more. We are all made to have purpose, to contribute, to serve, to help. And when we aren't doing those things, we become discontent, even when we're madly in love. So Rob and I set out to find someone to serve. We hopped a taxi and, in broken Spanish, asked the driver to take us to an orphanage. I don't know what we were thinking, but yes, we walked in the front door and asked if we could help. And for some reason, they let us.

There we were, playing with all these adorable kids on the playground, and then one fell. I ran over and picked the little guy up and wiped his tears. I held him and bounced him, and soon enough, he stopped crying and gave me a grin. Then a little girl started crying, so I put my new little friend down and ran over and picked her up. Then another kiddo started crying. Rob ran over to him, and then another kid cried, and another, and before you know it, the whole yard was crying, and Rob and I were running around, sweating, trying to comfort them, wishing we could cool off by a pool.

These kids weren't crying because they'd skinned their knees. They were crying because they had been abandoned and neglected, and all their little hearts wanted was someone to hold them and love them. They taught me what is true for all of us:

People are hurting and they want to be picked up in their pain.

Yes, it's hard work, and yes, running around carrying people and helping people and loving on people can be exhausting. But I'll tell you what . . . At the end of my life, do I want to look back and see the sweet vacations I went on and the nice things I got to enjoy? Or do I want to see myself doing more of what Jesus would do—running around, sweatin', picking up people in pain and telling them they matter?

The people who most inspire me are the ones who are running after hurting people, looking for opportunities to have *healing* collisions rather than wounded ones.

I think of my friend Lionel, who was heading into the grocery store when some drunk guy started hollering at him for money. As Lionel got closer, this guy said, "Cool shirt, man."

Lionel had things to do, but sensing God's Spirit might be ordaining this collision, he stopped and stood present with this guy who was numbing his pain, knowing Christ loved him. Lionel offered him his shirt. The guy declined, as if to be polite. Lionel offered again. The guy said, "In my culture we don't take, we trade."

Right there, Lionel took off his shirt and handed it to the man. The drunk man took off his dirty, alcohol-ridden shirt and handed it to Lionel, saying, "You might want to wash it. I've been wearing it for three days." Lionel put it on and walked right into the store, where he ran into my husband who was last-minute card shopping for Valentine's Day!

There's not a greater way that you and I can share Jesus' love than by taking off what is white as snow, hip and cool, and trading it for what is scarlet and alcohol stained.

I think of Pastor Jeff, whose church feeds homeless people every week. He also allows them to make their bed outside of his church each night, despite inconvenience and opinions. One morning I walked by him on my way to work as he hosed off the puke an unhoused man left for him to deal with. Jeff's light was brighter than the morning sun. He greeted me with humility and a smile that made him my new hero. He picked up the garbage, remains, and needles as we chatted. Pastor Jeff wouldn't be seen as an "influencer." He wouldn't be admired as a megachurch leader. But he pastors his city and the vulnerable people in it in a way that says, "You might have no home, you might have no family, but you have a place here."

I think of my friend Pam, who has given years of her life to serving men at a local family-home setting for adults living with HIV. Pam, a pastor's wife, took a lot of heat for doing this work but chose to keep showing up anyway, reminding these guys that they are loved and worthy. Her life has ushered so many precious men into a knowledge of Jesus' love because they saw hers first.

I think of a man I highly respect, a senior pastor who got fired for basically being "too old to be relevant." Now James shows up as a chaplain for people in crisis. He also facilitates funerals for the forgotten, people on the streets who pass away and no one seems to notice or care. This man, who could have easily decided to close the door to Jesus because Jesus' people hurt him, now opens the door for others to whom it has been closed.

I think of my surgeon friend Jim, who travels into the jungles of developing countries and performs surgeries on women with breast cancer. He could be kicking back in retirement but instead uses his education, his experience, his privilege, and his plenty to help those who would otherwise die. He goes out looking for places to shine his light—places that have no electricity, no hospitals, and no hope.

I think of my son Aidan, who chases down hurting people on the streets of our city. He started handing out cheeseburgers by himself on Sunday nights. No one knew he was doing it until the McDonald's drive-through guy asked what he did with fifty burgers at a time. When Aidan explained, the young man asked if he could come along. Now a swarm of students joins Aidan weekly, and their lives are being radically impacted while they impact others, one cheeseburger at a time.

I think of Kelly Welk, who found herself at an informational meeting about sex trafficking. She felt disturbed by the devastating stories, but she also felt ordinary, with no big talents or resources to make a difference. But Kelly asked, "What can I do?" She could host a great party. So she began hosting "freedom dinners" to raise awareness and funds, which led to the birth of Ciderpress Lane, an organization that now helps free women trapped in a life they did not choose.[1]

When we are staring a hurting world square in the eyes, feeling daunted by how to help, we can be inspired by Kelly and ask, "What can I do?" And you know what you can do . . . You can take some of that healed pain and go running after hurting people to bring healing. You've collided with Jesus. It's time.

Get off the bus.

Pick up some kids.

Trade your shirt.

Be family to people who've lost theirs.

Go visit the stranger.

Show up for people on their worst day.

Take your skills to the places and people who need them.

Hand out cheeseburgers.

Host beautiful dinners for beautiful causes.

Ask, "What can I do?" and then go do it.

21

the park bench

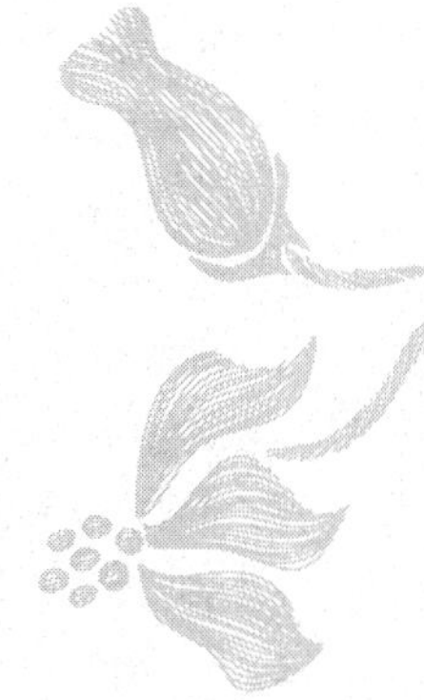

I was getting lunch for my kids before a soccer game. You know the kind, where the kids are like ten but the parents are acting like we're at the World Cup. Aidan, Bella, and I stopped at some podunk BBQ place, and while we were waiting, I checked my email. That's when I saw his name.

John.

My stomach fell to the ground. I hadn't talked to him in years. *How did he find me? What does he want?* Right there in the restaurant, while people were licking their greasy, BBQ-stained fingers, I started crying. When we got in the car, the kids asked what was wrong. I told them the man who had hurt me when I was a kid wanted to meet with me. I had heard he was battling a disease and was back to drinking again after being sober for many years, so maybe he wanted to talk before it was too late. Aidan said, "Mom, imagine wanting to be released of that burden." I cried even more. "I know, Aidan, I know."

I couldn't stop crying. I tried to get myself together for my kid's game. On the sidelines, I watched Bella, who was the very same age I was when I collided with this man. She was fragile, formative, beautiful. I could not imagine her having to face the fear I had to at that age. She was easy to mold and encourage and break and hurt. She was doing endless cartwheels, with her blonde hair flitting about. She was full of joy, optimism, naivete, and wild trust. I couldn't picture her feeling so anxious and alone. That day, she hugged me and comforted me with soft words of care and concern. I hugged her and comforted her that it was going to be OK because God was doing something.

Years and years of soul work had led to this collision. I wouldn't enter my ordinary patterns and run or move away or be busy. I knew what I would do without even having to pray.

Of course, I felt sickened by the idea. *What if this man hurts me again? What if he wants to get to me to get to my mom? What if he wants to make excuses for the past?* I ran through all the ways this could go bad. But this felt ordained, from God, like redemption was peeking through the cracks of my broken places. God does that, you know? God enters another hurt room in our heart and invites us to more healing. I knew the healing wasn't just for me. It would be for this man too.

It took me two days to respond. It wasn't a matter of *if* I would meet him, it was a matter of when I could muster up the courage.

We made plans to meet halfway, at Green Lake in Seattle, which meant a several-hour drive for each of us. I couldn't do it on my own, so Rob and the kids came. I needed the people who God used every day to remind me not only that redemption was possible but that redemption was my reality. Maybe it could be real here too. I needed their presence to remind me I was loved. I needed their courage when mine was jumping out of the car and changing its mind.

In my hyper state of anxiety that wanted to run and escape this, I begged of God, *What do You want me to say? Who do You want me to be?*

I heard God say, *Be Me.*

I wrote this down in my journal, as big as could be. I knew exactly what it meant. These might be two of the most powerful words you'll ever need, friend. When you don't know who to be, Jesus says, "Be Me." When you have to do something hard, Jesus says, "Be Me." When you have to face a fear or a fearmonger, Jesus says, "Be Me."

It had taken years of running into Jesus to prepare me for this moment. Who I was when I finally came face-to-face with this oppressor was who God had been shaping me to be. I would be like Jesus. I would collide with the man who had once terrorized us. And I knew with all my heart, this could be a new kind of collision.

My family and I waited in a coffee shop for this man I hadn't seen in decades. I was sure I would recognize him. I looked at every man in their sixties when they walked in. After fifteen minutes of staring at the wrong men, I saw him walk right up to my family, and for some crazy reason, I gave him the biggest hug you've ever seen. I surprised even myself. The compassion and love of God extended my arms around this man who had once afflicted me.

I introduced him to the loves of my life. Rob. Aidan. Bella.

My family went to play so that John and I could talk. We walked at a gentle pace toward the lake and sat on a park bench. We started with things like "Where do you live?" and "How are your kids?"

John was a frail shadow of the man I remembered. He began with, "An apology is not enough . . . I knew you were a whole person, and I didn't even treat you like a human being . . . I was a monster. You didn't deserve that . . . I have always cared about you . . . and what I did was so wrong . . ."

I was trying not to cry, but my eyes started raining years of pain. He said, "I was afraid you would cry." I tried to rein it in, but then I decided I would not protect him from my pain so that he could feel better about causing it. As breakable as he was, with great strength he owned up to the destruction, the abuse, the addiction, the pain. Admitting to the ways we have wounded others takes incredible courage. And I was sitting in his bravery.

When we own up and say out loud—

"I am sorry. You did not deserve what I did to you."

"I was hurting, and I did horrible things to hurt you."

"I've gone to a counselor to figure out how to talk to you."

—these all come from a place of strength that no weak, oppressive, abusive, power-mongering monster can display.

This kind of courage will find all of us sitting on park benches, having healing collisions, the kinds where we are left more whole than broken—the kinds that write stories of pain into stories of healing.

John and I had experienced a wounded collision years ago, and those wounds had hurt for years and years. We sat on that bench in need of a new kind of collision that would heal us both. And we were having it.

Jesus was there. He was sitting on that bench too.

I asked, "Why now? I'm in my forties." He explained that he was losing his faculties—his memory, his speech, his balance—and that the conversation he needed to have with me he would soon not be able to have. The timing of this conversation pointed toward how destined this moment was. He expressed a desire to be set free from the memories that chased him. I looked him in the eyes. Age had taken over and sickness was winning out. But even more, regret had begun to shrivel him. He wanted to be released, just like Aidan said.

Without falsehood, without pressure to be a certain way or say a certain Christian thing, I said, "You did hurt me. I still have a mess and leftovers from the pain. I still need healing, but God has begun that work in me. I can truly say that I don't have hatred or bitterness or anger toward you. I honor your heart to meet with me and own up to what you did. I want freedom for you."

And I said it. I said the thing I needed to say. The thing I could finally say and mean: "Be released into the peace God desires for you."

Somehow saying those words to him was like saying them to myself.

John had heard about Collide, the ministry I'd accidentally started, and that's how he had tracked me down. He asked about it, and I got to tell the story of how *our* wounded collision and many others had eventually led me to run into Jesus. And Jesus had met me in my pain, and He was using me to help other people in their pain.

He said, "Wow, I'm amazed."

"I am too," I said.

We hugged and said goodbye, and I watched him walk away, sure I would never see him again. I sat on that bench and waited for Rob and the kids. As soon as I saw them, I started sobbing. They ran to me and hugged me, and the frightened little girl in me cried and cried.

It is finished.

A chapter that had been hurting for a really long time was finally closed. My courage was finally greater than my fear. My forgiveness released my dreadful disdain. They flew away, never to be seen again. Jesus offered both of us the release we needed.

What God has been showing me my whole life is indeed true: Wounded people wound people. But I've also been learning: Healed people help heal people. The more healing we allow God to do in our lives, the more healing we can bring into the world. And boy, do we need it.

My family wrapped their arms around me and hugged me so hard that I just lost it. The three women across the walkway were taking pictures because they thought something epic was happening. Maybe something epic *was* happening. My kids spoke words of love over me. Rob was holding me and reminding me I was not alone. They covered me in prayers and engulfed me with their presence. I had a safe family. I was OK. I no longer needed to fear because fear had been replaced by peace. In all my pain, I had collided with Love, and that collision over and over again has been, and will continue to be, my lifeline to wholeness. And it can be yours too.

I don't know what park bench you might be called to sit on. Maybe God has called you to collide with someone who wounded you. Or maybe you are the one who needs to say you're sorry. Either way, if you don't know what to do, remember who you've been colliding with. Take cues from Him. You've run into Jesus, and you know who He is. You have begun to learn His moves, His way, His will. When you're scared, when you have to do something really hard, when He asks you to collide with pain and bring healing—remind yourself who you are called to be.

Beautiful Jesus says, "Be Me."

22

make it count

On the sidelines of our sons' football game, another mom said to me, "I want to make my cancer count." I realized that day that she watched the games differently than I did. Julia Pohlman watched them like she wasn't sure how many more she would get to watch. She loved her kids like crazy and surely wanted to watch them graduate and get married and grow old. She had been diagnosed with stage 4 cancer, and it had spread into her breasts, lungs, and even her spine.

Julia's response to her diagnosis was "Could I lie in bed all day? Yes, but that's not living with cancer, that's dying from it." This attitude led her to start an organization in the midst of her fight called Team Julia, which has been helping fund cancer research and assisting other cancer patients with their hospital bills.[1] Julia ended up saying goodbye to her children and her husband and is now living in the perfect place, where there is no more cancer and no more goodbyes.

At her funeral, a lot of the boys on the county champ football team showed up in their green-and-white jerseys just to say to their friend who had lost his mother, "We are on your team in victory and in loss." Sitting in the waft of "It Is Well with My Soul" and hearing countless stories of this woman who had lived her entire life for Jesus, I witnessed so many people being invited to live like she did, like her Lord did. Julia invited us into something we *all* want: to make our lives count, even the painful parts.

It is inevitable that you and I will crash right into pain whether we like it or not. Jesus Himself told us, "In this world you will have trouble."[2] As much as we want to, we can't run from hardship, but we can choose what we do with it. The people who most inspire me are the people who are purposing their pain. They are the people who say, "If I have to undergo this suffering, if I have to live this chapter, if I have to experience this grief, I will make my pain count for other people's healing."

I shared with you a little bit about Christine, who was in the Wounded Collision Bible Study that met in my living room years ago. She was the one who was in that horrific accident when a young child was killed, through no fault of her own. I walked alongside sweet Christine for years as she agonized over the death of that child. There were no words or prayers that could take away the pain, no theology to calm it. This kind of traumatic event starts to mess with your sense of safety and security and your belief that God is good. Christine was afflicted by the fear that something terrible might happen unexpectedly. This anxiety started paralyzing her decisions, her job, her travels, and her dreams. But this brave young woman recognized the need for healing. She allowed our group to support her, and she regularly met with a therapist, which felt like God's hand grabbing hers to get the help she needed.

Simultaneously, Collide began to grow. The more we handed out permission slips for women to be real about their hurts, the more women were being real. And the need was overwhelming. After our events, I found myself meeting with women for up to eight hours a day. Women were coming out of the woodwork, opening up about their grief, infertility, sexual assault, religious baggage, affairs, self-esteem issues, eating disorders, suicidal ideations, and on and on. Boy, someone should have warned me what would happen when we told people God could handle pain and heal it. I could point them to Jesus, but I knew they needed more than I could give them. They needed professionals better equipped to help with trauma, mental health diagnoses, substance abuse, and crisis intervention.

These college-aged girls and I were blown away by how God was meeting us in our brokenness and using us to meet others in theirs. Christine was grieving and doing the work of healing with God while also serving these women coming to Collide. Together, we watched what God was doing with all our pain.

Christine received a large settlement from the accident. She didn't want it. The money could do nothing to take away the pain or make the loss of a child ever be OK. She agonized over its lack of redemption. She and her husband prayed separately, and they both sensed God telling them to give a portion of the money to Collide to help start a counseling program. Over the years, this program has helped thousands of women take the brave step to get help and healing—women like the mom on meth and the girl who couldn't stop crying after her ex-boyfriend took his own life. Their lives have changed because Christine chose to purpose her pain for the healing of others.

That is what our Lord did with His own life and what He can do with ours.

The night before Jesus died, He broke bread and gave thanks, saying, "This is My body, broken for you, and this is My blood, poured out for you."[3] Jesus gave thanks not because He liked being mocked, spat on, and whipped. He was thankful for the wholeness God would usher in because of His brokenness. Jesus was thankful for what God could do with pain. If God could purpose *His* pain, He can surely purpose ours. He can purpose your tears. He can purpose your past. He can purpose your failure.

Does it mean you'd choose to go through the pain all over again? No. But you can choose to allow something healing to come out of something hard.

You might be acquainted with the five stages of grief as defined by Elisabeth Kübler-Ross, a Swiss psychiatrist: denial, anger, bargaining, depression, and acceptance.[4] David Kessler, another grief expert, has since added a sixth stage as a result of his own loss: finding meaning.

Kessler lost his twenty-one-year-old son, and he says, "I knew I couldn't and wouldn't stop at acceptance. There had to be something more." He teaches, "Loss is simply what happens to you in life. Meaning is what *you* make happen."[5] Kessler became a grief counselor, speaker, and author and has found great meaning in turning his loss into a way to bring comfort to others.

I don't know what making meaning out of your pain and grief might look like for you, but sometimes it looks like writing your feels and sharing them with other people on a similar journey. Sometimes it means starting a scholarship fund in your loved one's name. Sometimes it looks like going into a field of work to help people you now have empathy and compassion for. Sometimes it looks like coming alongside kids in a mentoring role because you so wish you'd had that when you were young. Sometimes it looks like serving at the food bank because you waited in those long lines for too many years yourself. Sometimes it looks like taking your anger and your grief and painting your guts out for other people to behold. And sometimes it looks like opening your home to people in need of family because you know what that's like. Sometimes it looks like advocating for victims of abuse because you have been one. I don't know what making meaning looks like for you, but I do know that when you're doing it, you'll know. You'll feel that meaning deep in your soul, and it will help heal you.

We can't go back and rewrite our story. But you know what we can do? We can purpose our pain. We can make it count. We can allow our pain to bring someone else healing. And I have found that *we* gain more healing too.

A few years ago, I sat at my mother's bedside in a hospital for nearly a month. She had all sorts of issues, including an infectious disease that threatened to be fatal. She was a shell of who she had been. Rob was amazing and stood by my side the whole month. Dad called and checked in often. Funny how Mom and Dad always wanted good for each other even though they didn't want each other. I was grateful for the support. There was talk of power of attorney, a code was called . . . It was all so upsetting.

One day, I took a break from the hospital and got a bit lost on some country road. I was searching for coffee, but what I really needed was God. I was keenly aware that my mom might not make it, and I was broken up over her life, our life. I wanted the story to write differently than it had.

When I returned, I sat next to her in the ICU. I wept and pleaded, advocated and grieved. I held her hands, and like I did as a little girl, I massaged her back, writing letters in a message she could feel . . .

I L O V E Y O U

All I had ever wanted since I was a little girl was her wholeness. And yet here we were, broken as could be.

We can wish our story had been written differently. Or we can begin to see that even in the pain—even *because of* the pain—we have experienced beauty and good, meaning and compassion, healing and redemption. Because of the pain, we have gained empathy, wisdom, perseverance, surrender, faith, insight, story.

I looked at my mom's time-wrinkled hands, her skin that I had watched age to a reddish purple. She smelled like hospital, no longer like Oil of Olay. She slept, her body fighting hard to live. Even in this pain, I was overwhelmed by God's goodness.

I always wanted a life without this woundedness, but I now see how God has used it all. I understand what it feels like to be abandoned and neglected, but I also understand what it feels like to be picked up, adopted, chosen, and held. I have felt the touch of God, the healing of God, the restoration of God. I know deep within my soul, now, that I am loved and worthy and that our God is good. And all He ever wanted was to chase down my mom and me to tell us so. So, I could sit in a hospital room and feel the ache for her life and for parts of mine, but I could also praise God for saving me and using my pain to help save and heal others. Pain has shaped me, refined me, taught me, humbled me, and found me, over and over again needing a Healer and finding Him.

So I'm with Julia. I want my life and my pain to count. Seeing that God can take hardship and turn it into something healing—that feels a little like heaven's come down to earth. And don't you want that? Don't you crave deep down in your soul for something good, something redemptive, something healing to come out of so much hard? Make it count, friend. Make it count.

23
always

Whittle down what's most important to God, and Jesus makes it pretty clear: It's love. He said: "'Love the Lord your God with all your heart and with all your soul and with all your mind.' This is the first and greatest commandment. And the second is like it: 'Love your neighbor as yourself.'"[1] We're called to always love, but it isn't always easy. Yet we cannot get out from under the call to love even if we try.

Love is not easy when we have to love someone we don't even like. It's not easy when our neighbors build their fence on our property line, or when their dogs poo in our yard and we're expected to pick it up. Love is not easy when the mean girl is bullying our kid and her mom does nothing about it. Love is not easy when our spouse is addicted to porn or when our teenagers groan and demand rides and food and money. Love is not easy when a stranger gets confrontational or when a person with different political opinions pops off at our dinner table. Love is not easy when our mother-in-law tells us what we are doing for Thanksgiving or when Uncle Ted drinks himself into a stupor on Christmas. And it's especially not easy when we are faced with loving someone we have spent most of our life hating.

Mom called . . . John was moving in.

You can imagine my shock. They hadn't talked in ages, and I hadn't talked to him since the park bench two years prior. He had expressed how hurt he had been by my mother, and now he was moving in? He and I had made our peace, and apparently that and my mom almost dying in the hospital had caused him to want to make peace with her too.

He was moving back in thirty years after we had moved out.

"I don't know why you're so surprised," Mom said on the other end of the line.

"Mommmm!! You're skipping right to the moving-in-together part without explaining the peace, forgiveness, and reconciliation story??"

Great. A pair of aging and ailing alcoholics with a toxic, abusive past, who have damaged so many of their relationships and now have only each other to rely on. How in the world would they not become who they used to be—two lost souls drowning their wounds in box wine and denial?

It was a recipe for disaster, and we had all tried cooking it before. I was annoyed and triggered and all the things. Could my mother not make a freakin' good decision to save her life? I mean, this made no sense.

"It will help us both out," she reasoned. "He will help pay rent, and I can help cook for him because he needs care. I need you and Rob to come help me get his room ready."

What a nightmare. She expected me not only to buy in wholeheartedly but to help make it happen.

You're right, I did forgive him. I had released him into the arms of God on that park bench. But I didn't sign up to spend Christmases with him. I didn't sign up to become family again. I didn't sign up to *serrrrve* him.

Her outright dismissal of the fact that this was a man who had harmed us was maddening. She didn't ask how I felt. She didn't wonder if I would feel comfortable visiting him with the kids. It was her, once again, acting like what happened hadn't happened. It was like her years of being blackout drunk made her forget reality, and I was supposed to forget too.

The next thing I knew, I was face-to-face with these two people who had wrecked me. I walked into the house, and there they were, sitting on my childhood hippie-kid bed in the middle of my mother's living room—the bed that he had once broken. I couldn't believe the hauntedness of it all. But here they were, casually talking to me about where to find the cleaning supplies.

Love is not a thing you muster up because that's what good little Christians do. Love is not a rule we follow like we follow the speed limit. Love is not proper etiquette, like putting your napkin on your lap and eating with your mouth closed so people don't judge you. Love is not like paying taxes . . . something you have to do or else. Love is not something you can fake. Lord knows, we don't actually love annoying people because we feel guilty and obligated. And we don't love family because we share their DNA. Jesus knew that we don't actually love hard-to-love people because our pastor told us to.

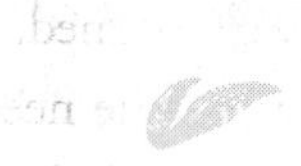

I was studying a Bible passage on love one afternoon, trying to unpack it for a message I had to preach. And wouldn't you know it, on my way to the public restroom, I ran right into one of those women from the cool kids club. Pretending to be nice, I said, "Heyyyy, Suzy Q!" Her friend joked, "Wow! First and last name? Sounds like she's in trouble."

I was caught red-handed. Triggered, I had acted out of pain rather than love. And her friend had seen it. It was like all my truth left the building. That's what happens sometimes when we run into people who hurt us. It's like we time travel, and there we are in the past, being hurt all over again. Almost as though all the healing God has done vanishes. In the space of a second, we forget who we are and who they are. We know God loves us, and we know God loves them, but for some reason, we don't act like it. The old pain threatens to steal our center. The work isn't to pretend we don't lose our grounding in God's love. The work is to get it back.

I walked into the bathroom and heard God say, *Whyyyy donnnn't you love her?*

Right there in the stall, it hit me, so I told Him. God and I do a lot of talking over pee. It hurt to admit, but it felt so dang real. *I don't love her because she triggers everything in me that believes I'm unlovable.* I finally realized what is true for all of us: The degree to which we love has everything to do with how loved we believe we are.

The work of loving others isn't manufacturing some fake, cheesy, inauthentic, robotic, rule-oriented act. The work of loving others begins with allowing God's love to penetrate all the places and spaces within us that don't yet believe they are lovable.

We can be frustrated with our need for *more* healing and find ourselves like, *Really Jesus, I need to run back to You, again?*

And we can sense His response wrapped in welcome, *Yes, kiddo, again.*

The Bible says, "We love because he first loved us."[2] Our ability to love others is in direct proportion to our ability to receive God's love for us. Maybe that's why we've been flopping at loving when it's not easy. We've been trying to love from a place other than love: fear, insecurity, control, guilt, penance, selfishness, desperation, or duty. You can't love out of these places. You can only love out of Love. Scripture says love "comes from God." God is the origin of love. In fact, "God is love."[3] We have to go to the Source to draw love. You can't produce it by yourself. You can't pretend it into existence.

Is there someone you are being asked to love or serve and, like me, you don't want to? Do you have a family member who causes most of your anxiety and who, if you're honest, you don't even like, let alone love? Do you have a friend you can't even fake loving right now?

Here's the deal. If you are taking inventory and you recognize you aren't loving like you want to, consider this an indicator light on your dashboard. It's showing you that you've lost sight of how loved you are. If your warning light is going off, this is not the moment to put on the gas and pretend you've got love when you don't. It's the moment to take a trip to the Source of love. And when you get full on His love, you will overflow to the point that you can't help but love people who are hard to love. It won't be just one moment though. The more trips we take back to God to be loved, the more loving we become.

You and I have journeyed together, and we have seen the compassion and the grace and the goodness of God. Over and over, we have watched Him collide with and love other people. And that's just the thing: It's easy to believe other people are loved and so hard to believe *we* are. And yet Jesus showed us just how much He loved us with His life and in His death.

Friend, God chose to crash into earth for you. His love experienced people talking about Him behind His back for you. It was mocked for you. His love felt pain and suffering, rejection and abandonment for you. It entered the broken human experience for you. His love took on everything that has ever made you feel unlovable. It wore wounds on the cross for you. God crashed right into all this mess and made Himself fully vulnerable for you.

The very definition of the word *vulnerable* is "capable of being wounded or hurt."[4] Jesus didn't run from pain. Nope, this God we say we follow, this God we say we wanna be like, His love hurts Him.

C. S. Lewis says, "To love at all is to be vulnerable. Love anything, and your heart will certainly be wrung and possibly be broken. If you want to make sure of keeping it intact, you must give your heart to no one, not even to an animal. Wrap it carefully round with hobbies and little luxuries; avoid all entanglements; lock it up safe in the casket or coffin of your selfishness. But in that casket—safe, dark, motionless, airless—it will change. It will not be broken; it will become unbreakable, impenetrable, irredeemable."[5]

You know why it's so dang hard to love wounded people? Because we want to protect ourselves from getting hurt. We want to lock ourselves up to stay safe. We want to avoid more hardship.

To love is to be vulnerable.

It will hurt. Just like it hurt Jesus. And yes, you have experienced too much pain. And I know you don't want more. And yes, you can build taller walls, and you can shut down, and you can run away, and you can hide in closets. But you can't love from a closet, protecting yourself from pain. And you can't heal there either.

I never saw serving John as being a chapter in my story. And I certainly never wanted to feel a vulnerability that left me looking weak or inferior, defenseless or susceptible to him ever again. And nothing will make you feel that way more than holding a mop.

But there I was, hauling mattresses and furniture, doing what was expected. Not because I'm awesome. Not because I owed them anything. Not because God guilted me. But because God gutted me.

I carried the cleaning supplies into the bedroom and vacuumed every square inch.

God felt the suffering of laying Himself down for those who hurt Him.

God felt being wronged and the death of having to let go of being right.

God loves us so.

I swept the cobwebs in the corners of the room.

God felt the agony of serving those who knew not what they were asking.

God felt the nakedness of showing kindness to those who violently lashed out at Him.

God loves us so.

I dusted and cleaned the window.

God felt the pain of mockery that says, "This kind of love is cowardly."

God felt the vulnerability that exposes itself to getting hurt.

God loves us so.

A tidal wave of Jesus came over me while I was cleaning. I was so sure, more than anything in that moment, that God's love is for me, but it is also for them.

Jesus loves Mom and John. He never wanted them to be hurt. And it was their hurt that hurt me. And right there in that room with Windex in hand—looking like I like to clean, like I'm freaking Mother T over here when we all know I'm not—all I wanted was to give this man who had hurt me a comfy room to call home. All I wanted was for them to know this Love. Oh, if they only knew this Love.

This was a new kind of collision, and that's what happens when we let God love us. He breaks into the dark corners of our hearts and does what we never could.

I'm right here with you trying to figure out this love thing. My runs to the Source are changing me. And they'll change you too. You'll run right into someone who hurt you, and all you need to do to get grounded is run right to Jesus. Let Him love you from the inside out. When you are sure of nothing else more than you are sure of this one thing—Jesus loves *you*—then you will be able to love even the people who wounded you most.

God breaks into closets and counseling offices. God breaks into broken families and broken friendships. He breaks into generational sin, addiction, and abuse. And He can use you to be a part of all this healing. But first, you have to let His love break into *you*. Once you know you are always loved, you will love always. Let God break into your life, your heart, and your inability to love and be loved, and He will do something more powerful, more healing, and more beautiful than you could ever imagine.

24

the yellow butterflies

My mom became obsessed with green burials. Of course Mom pressed into this environmentally conscious approach with no toxins, chemicals, concrete, or coffin. She took a class and gave us books with pictures of dead people. It wasn't like she talked about it once—it was every time we were together.

Mom was starting to read my writing online and to send me Bob Dylan's. She started asking questions about Jesus. Mom had never talked about faith or Jesus in a curious way, so this was new territory. She wanted to talk about how people's lives were being changed by me sharing my story. She was starting to see that God was using my pain to help others in theirs, even though she never wanted to talk about my hurt or what had caused it. She told me I should write this book. I told her it would be hard for both of us. She got emotional and said that if it could help people, I should do it. "Besides," she said, "you're really good at writing." I knew Mom was just being a mom, believing in her kid. I also knew that telling our story would hurt, but it would heal too.

She was aging and, I think, scared, though she never said it. I don't think Mom knew how to work out on the outside what was going on inside. I don't think she knew how to reconcile things, how to do "I'm sorrys," how to express a desire for connection—or share the regrets that had wrecked it. What she did know was that her day would come, like it does for all of us. And what she hoped for most was to spend as many of her last days with us as possible.

Keep in mind my mother wasn't dying. Our visits about death were a real downer. She bought a grave plot and wanted us to come see it. Nothing in me thought it was a good idea to take teenagers and go hang out at a cemetery. I mean, you can't even get them excited about ice cream with the parents. How was I going to get them stoked about dead people? Sometimes we have to honor people in weird ways. So that's what we did. We drove a few hours away to my mom's future cemetery.

As soon as we got there, Mom started talking to the kids about her body returning to the dirt and worms. She wanted us to have fun at her funeral and drop silly things on her. "Dirt and worms. Dirt and worms," she kept saying.

I was upset. This hope my mom had really bothered me. I don't want to just become dirt and worms, and I don't want you to either. I don't want to say goodbye to my family and never see them again. And I didn't want my mom to have experienced so much pain just to become compost. I wanted more.

There is a path from the cemetery to a cliff with the most drop-dead gorgeous view of the ocean. Rob, Aidan, and Bella walked ahead with Mom. I hung back and walked with John. Somehow, in those last few years, every time I was with him, a compassion overtook me that I knew wasn't mine.

He was frail and weak, and a slight divot in the path could send him tripping. He had no aggression left in him, more passivity. No more overpowering strength, just weakness. No confidence, mostly fear. I owed him nothing, and I knew that. But Jesus gave him everything, and I knew that too.

As we walked the gravel road toward the bluff, yellow butterfly after yellow butterfly after white fluttered past, as if to brag about the great, great possibility of such beauty coming out of a caterpillar.

And I heard God say, *I am a God of the butterfly.*

It was like He was assuring me, *I am a God who can change life, transform life, resurrect life. I am a God who can create something out of nothing. I am a God who can breathe life into dust. I made the flower bulb that endures the winter and then blossoms in absolute brilliance in spring. I endured death on a cross, was buried in a grave, and rose up, and when I did, I said, "Enough with dirt and worms."*

Dirt and worms have no hold on Me. And dirt and worms have no hold on you.

We reached the edge and saw the bright blue sky, flaunting clouds that spoke of an Artist, a Maker, a Creator, One who made a world where butterflies are possible, metamorphosis is possible, rebirth is possible, resurrection is possible.

Rob told me later that my mom had expressed to him on that walk that she would like to stop drinking. Mom had *never* owned up to her alcohol problem. Rob had always been so good to her. He had served her over the years despite how much pain she had caused me. He had built her deck, fixed her appliances, gotten her jobs, and cleaned his plate with a beaming smile after one of her home-cooked meals. He didn't have the baggage with her that I did. He spoke logic into her wild, harebrained ideas. And every once in a while, this whimsy-wanderer took his advice.

My mom had been extremely vulnerable with Rob that day. To express a desire to change is huge. She had asked him not to tell me, but of course he did. I think Mom knew the likelihood of her actually doing it was miracle-status impossible, and she hadn't wanted to get my hopes up. Of course I wanted to hold on to hope, but I had also become an expert at talking myself out of hope. We do that. Those who've been disappointed by hope—we become really good at keeping hope under wraps. Maybe you can relate. Maybe you are in hope management too?

John ended up breaking his hip that year and moving into a care facility. And Mom went downhill after that, isolated during the pandemic, and—I am sure—drinking herself into oblivion. She sold her house and moved closer to us so we could help her more, but far enough away that I didn't have to deal with her drinking on the daily.

Almost exactly a year after we had walked in the cemetery together, my mom died unexpectedly.

Her need to numb her pain finally caught up to her. We said goodbye to Mom as she had requested, green burial and all. The invite list was small—about twenty of us, dogs included.

Our family of four drove up to the cemetery and parked. I saw the dirt pile and the hearse and started to panic. I didn't want to see her body. I didn't want to see a hole. I didn't want any of it. I went for a walk away from the others. I was so desperate for God to meet me, and as Hallmark cheesy as it sounds, I whispered back to the God who had met me there a year prior, "God please just show me a butterfly."

And wouldn't you know it . . . a white butterfly flittered past me just like I needed it to.

We all wore colorful clothes and wacky glasses. Mom would have loved it. As each person my mom had loved arrived, I placed a lei around their neck. Alongside her silhouetted body, lying so vulnerable on the ground next to the open grave, we told honest stories about my crazy mother. One of my aunts started to share, and as she talked about the one and only Kimothy, a butterfly landed on her shirt. I secretly gasped.

My other aunt got on her knees in the grass. She patted down her sister's arms and legs and then hugged her and kissed her forehead. She let her goodbye be covered in love, and the years of withdrawal and regret, guilt and ache felt wisped away in grace and forgiveness.

After each person shared beautiful, whimsical, tragic tales of my mother's life, we sprinkled confetti into the grave, just as she had hoped.

My Hawaiian friend Ron, who Mom had really liked, played a Bruddah IZ song for her and "Amazing Grace" for me. Each person placed their lei on her body, and then I placed a crown of flowers on my sweet mama's head.

I wept over our shared life of pain, feeling unable to catch my breath and control myself for the others. I felt a hand on my shoulder.

It was my dad.

He stood behind me and whispered, "I am here with you, Willow."

Through many dangers, toils, and snares,
I have already come;
'Tis grace hath brought me safe thus far,
And grace will lead me home.

The Lord has promised good to me,
His Word my hope secures;

He will my Shield and Portion be,
As long as life endures.[1]

I looked up, and wouldn't you know it, butterflies swept over my mom's body, and then we lowered her into the dirt and worms.

The God of the butterfly showed up for me that day. Though I couldn't see it when I was younger, I now see He has been showing up for me my entire life. He does that, you know? He collides with us over and over again, proving He can bring beauty out of pain, and so there I was and here I am. All I can see is dirt and worms, but I'm counting on God to be more than all I can see.

Dirt and worms won't have the last word. My power and resurrection have the last word.

Have you longed for a healing that is yet to be healed? Have you prayed for something one trillion times and it's still horribly broken? Have you wondered where this Jesus is when all you've needed was for Him to show up and do the one thing you long for most? I know this pain too. I didn't get my miracle. I got other miracles, but not the one I wanted, the one I had wished for since I was a little girl, every time I blew out my birthday candles. And maybe you haven't gotten your miracle. Might I remind us that we are people of faith in the not yet. We are a people who hold hope for what we cannot see.

I cannot wait to see my mom whole in heaven. I hope for it with all the faith I have. Hebrews says faith is being sure about what we hope for and certain about what we don't see.[2] And though I can't be certain of a heaven where my mom dances free, though I can't see her healed, I wholeheartedly believe in a God who does all that He can to rescue us from our pain and sorrow, even unto our very last breath. So I hope and wait earnestly to see my mom no longer needing to numb her pain, no longer thirsty, no longer hurting. I believe in a

God who loves the likes of her, whose grace abounds so big I cannot comprehend it, who gives broken, hurting people a second chance in a stunning eternity where there are no more tears.

So if you need a friend to hope with, I'm her. I'm waiting in the not yet. I need more than death and dirt. I need a God who triumphs over death and mocks the enemy. I need a God who can usher in new life out of what has gotten so, so old. I need a God who can take this side of heaven and make it look like a beautiful redemption story that goes into forever.

We might feel like all we see is death and dirt and worms, but we have a God who whispers, *I can transform what seems over, insignificant, unlikely, and broken into something magical, something that dances like a canvas in the sky, capturing the attention of all who gaze upon it. I will usher in a hope you cannot see, a healing you cannot see, and a new life you cannot see.*

You just wait. I'm the God of the butterfly.

25

mended and restored

My Cindy died. She was like family to me, a spiritual mother if you will. Before I could catch a breath, my mother died a week later. Losing them within days of each other leveled me.

Just an hour or so after I found out about my mom's sudden death, I walked into her apartment and fell to pieces. Her essence was in the room, the last time I would have it. Her ice pack was still melting. Her blood drops on the floor. Her morning coffee cup, drying next to the sink. I was overcome by our story, our shared pain, the deep-cutting regret, by how I wished it had gone versus how it went.

My mom . . . was gone. The ache of hoping she hadn't died alone and the weight of her loneliness felt heavier than I could bear. Our *we* was now just me. I sat there on her bed, and Bella held me as I came undone.

"Lorrrrd, why was she so, so hard to love?" I wailed. "Why was I so awwwwful at it? Why did it goooo this waaaay?"

I was as broken as I've ever been and beating myself up that I hadn't done more. Regret likes to be the first visitor to show up in grief. *I should have spent more time with her. I shouldn't have pushed her away. I should have been more loving.* My daughter comforted me as I ugly grieved my mother. All I could do was hope God could enter this agony that was threatening to wreck me. And He showed up in one of the most powerful ways I have ever experienced.

A sharp sense woke me from wailing, and I knew I was supposed to see something in that room. Rob was rummaging through Mom's stuff to find the paperwork the hospital had requested. I walked aimlessly over to her desk and then sat back down, exhausted and scared of what thumbing through her belongings might do to me. I noticed my mom's recycling, and I instantly knew that I was supposed to look in that box. I pulled out bills, junk mail, and to-do lists. And I kept finding . . .

receipt
after receipt
after receipt
for alcohol.

Bella laid out the receipts by purchase date. The bed was covered. My mother was buying a bottle of vodka and a bottle of wine every two days, consuming them alone. My mother's denial was still alive, already spinning lies, blaming me. And it was right there in that anguished room that God so sweetly showed up to insist, *This is your truth.* This *was why she was so, so very hard to love.*

The ER doctor had alluded that there might be more to my mom's death, and now I wanted to know. We called the doctor and learned that my mom had been at a hospital the month prior, showing signs of pulmonary issues due to alcoholism. But my mother had told them she rarely drank.

Here again, God was so graciously reminding me what was real, since my mom had been playing pretend for so very long. The truth was my mom had ultimately died from trying to numb her pain. And here I was, left with so much need for healing.

My mother had needed restoration her entire life but had always seemed to push it away. After her death, I needed restoration and knew my mom's life would remind me not to do the same.

You and I, we have a Restorer, and He will show up in our pain over and over again. He will show up when we are raw and messy and absolutely soul-crushed broken. He shows up there like only He can, and He will begin to restore what needs mending, but *only* if we allow it.

In Matthew 12, Jesus offered restoration to a man who longed for it, but it seemed as though he had all kinds of reasons to push it away.[1] Before we turn the page on this story, we have to know that this was the Sabbath, and some Jesus haters were making this moment all about Jesus breaking laws rather than about Him healing pain.

Work was forbidden on the Sabbath, but so many man-made rules had been added to define work. They included carrying a "burden," which was anything that weighed as little as two figs. You could be condemned to death for having sex with your spouse, shopping, drawing water, lighting a fire, or catching a fish. It was a burden just to remember what was considered a burden.[2] It was believed that if you kept these commandments, you kept the law of God, and if you didn't, you broke it. This belief was so intense that even if an enemy attacked you and your family on the Sabbath, you were to let yourselves be slaughtered.[3] The Pharisees created so many burdens, misunderstandings, wounds, distrust, toxic theology, and God-slander that people who needed God's help were left pushing Him away.

Jesus gave them a piece of His mind with a "You talk big for a bunch of hypocrites. You would save an animal but not your neighbor." Then He turned to this man whose hand did not work and said, "Stretch out your hand."[4] Imagine being this guy. If you wouldn't fight to save your family on the Sabbath, you certainly wouldn't say yes to the offer of healing. Restoration was standing right in front of him, and like us, he had so many understandable reasons to push it away.

We get it—accepting help and healing might cause more harm. *If I do what God is asking, they might get angry. If I go to a counselor, something might come up I don't want coming up. If I tell my spouse I have this problem, they might leave. If I quit drinking, I will feel the pain.* The fear that healing might be uncomfortable, hard, or painful keeps us broken and longing to be whole.

This man could have thought, *It's just a shriveled hand.* We do that, you know? *It's just anxiety. It's just diabetes. It's just an occasional pill. It's just a fight. It's just something* . . . until it's just so much more. It's just a shriveled hand until it's a shriveled capacity, a shriveled spirituality, a shriveled self-esteem. We make our pain small and insignificant, and when we do, we fend off mending and restoration.

This man also had every reason not to trust Jesus, especially if Jesus was like these hurtful religious people. And we get that. Love could be standing right in front of us, and we would push it away because the people who were supposed to love us hurt us. We keep God and God's people at a distance because their help has felt harmful. We might know we need help and helpers, love and Love, but we turn them away. And we are left to find our own cure.

We also push restoration away because we assume, *I have to heal me*, or, *God has to heal me*. One of these puts too much power on self, and the other removes all agency and participation. This guy was probably afraid to stretch out his hand. He was most likely hoping Jesus would do for him what He did for the blind, the mute, the lame. We are like that. We want the abracadabra, to have our name on the prayer chain, and to be the miracle people prayed for. And yeah, sometimes God does that. But sometimes He asks *us* to move, to act, to engage in the very healing we know we need.

All I had ever wanted was for my mother to quit drinking. I hadn't understood why she never did, and after she died, the need for an answer was killing me. God was inviting me to participate in my own healing again.

Again?

Again.

God led me to an addiction specialist named Pippa. In our first session, in a British accent, she dropped multiple f-bombs and just as much truth, and my soul felt like it was being stitched up word by word. I was begging to understand why my mom had never gotten restoration. Pippa was honest: "You wanted your mom's recovery more than *she* wanted it."

Agonized, I said, "I don't get it—did she not know she had a problem? Her drinking gave up her only kid . . . How could she not know she needed healing? Why didn't she quit to get me back? Did she not see how her whole life her alcoholism had distanced her from her sisters, her grandkids, her friends, me?"

The specialist said, "Oh, she knew she had a problem. The mantra of an addict is . . .

I have a problem, but not today . . .

I'll deal with it soon . . .

Someday . . .

But not today."

And I got it. I finally understood my mom, because I understood this mantra. My mom had hurt from all the pain she'd experienced as a kid, all the pain she'd caused me as a kid. Getting well would have meant feeling all that pain. And she just couldn't bear it. Mom had known she'd needed healing.

Not today.

Someday.

I've said "someday" myself. And I bet you have too. When Jesus said, "Stretch," He was asking this man to participate in his own healing *right now*. And He asks the same of you and me.

A few months after my mom passed, my friend Misha asked how I was doing, and I shared everything I was learning from Pippa. I told her that I finally *got* my mom. I understood why she hurt, why she had never gotten well, and why I now realized it'd had nothing to do with me.

Misha looked at me and said, "I'm blown away, Willow."

"What do you mean?" I asked, not grasping what she was seeing.

"Your mom is dead, and you're still trying to figure out how to love her."

Not for one second had I thought that seeking help in my grief was me trying to love my mom. I was hurting and needed healing, so I went chasing after it. And what I found was unexpected. The more I stretched toward Jesus for healing, the more I loved the person who had wounded me the most. The more I loved the person who'd wounded me the most, the more I healed.

Here I was, with my mama gone.

And I was *finally* able to fully love her.

And *feel fully loved by her*.

I was overcome by this entire journey, by God's goodness to me, by His healing.

When my mother knocked on my door years ago, I ran to avoid her. But our good, beautiful, gracious God met me there. And He invited me to do the craziest thing ever:

Run into pain.

Running into pain is the only way to get the healing we long for. My mom didn't want to feel pain. Neither do I, and neither do you. And neither did this man colliding with Jesus. But Jesus invited him to stretch out his hand anyway. This could hurt. This could have repercussions. But right there in the middle of a crowd of haters, the man with the shriveled hand risked healing. The Bible says, "He stretched it out and it was completely restored, just as sound as the other."[5]

This man's healing caused quite a stir. In fact, it was the thing that set the Pharisees off to plot Jesus' death. Jesus knew they would use this miracle against Him, but He chose to heal this man anyway. This man's healing could have waited a day. The consequences could have been avoided. But Jesus said, "Oh no. Your healing is worth the risk."

Jesus says *Today*.

Today I want to heal the thing that holds you back.

Today I want you to stop numbing your pain.

Today we're going to do battle with your insecurities.

Today you're going to give up all self-harm.

Today you're going to surrender.

Today you're going to let the light in.

Today you're going to call for help.

Today you're going to say yes to trusting again.

Today you're going to pour out the bottles.

Today you're going to bring Me your pain.

Friend, do not say *someday* when Jesus says *today*.

You can keep rain checking your own restoration, but Jesus doesn't put off to tomorrow what He can start healing right now.

Right after my mom passed, I spoke to hundreds of women at a conference, calling them to say yes to healing *today*. Women in tears, desperate for help, regretful, hungry, and inspired that a new story might be possible walked to the front because they finally felt like they weren't alone. And they aren't. If there's one thing I've learned, it's that we *all* hurt and we all long for healing. The line of hurting women included two teenagers in black hoodies and dark eyeliner who told me how hard life had been since the mother of one of them had passed away. Another woman bawled, saying her husband had told her that very night that she was trash and would never amount to anything.

And then a woman who reeked of alcohol came up to me and said, "I'm your mom."

I had just shared about the pain of my mother's addiction and the healing God was doing. This lady was crying and said, "Tonight I realized the pain I've caused my daughters. I have never thought about the damage my alcoholism has caused for them until now. I don't wanna die like your mom. I don't wanna do that to my babies."

She called her adult daughters the next morning and apologized for a lifetime of pain.

I had waited for a call like that my whole life.

The next week, I spent an evening handing this woman black coffee to keep down the shakes. In the past I would have run from "my mom," but here I was, breathing in the smell of wine coming out of her pores. This woman's bloodshot eyes, red face, and tremoring hands threatened my hope that she would get sober. She paced like her life was on the line. This was going to go one of two ways, and she knew either would hurt.

She was almost preaching to me, proclaiming the God she knew and the addiction she hated. She knew she could keep saying "someday," but my story was living proof that she needed to say "today." Every time she looked at me, she saw her own daughters, the ones her wounds had wounded. She couldn't go back and erase what she'd done. But she could let God write a new story. This woman was having a collision with Jesus that was wrecking her life in a good way.

She left me five bajillion voicemails in the days before she flew out to rehab, and I have all of them saved on my phone. She was emotional, she was desperate, she was hopeful, and she was drunk. But she was going to get help. She did what I had always wanted my mom to do. And crazy enough, my mom's pain helped her do it. She told her girls they were worth it. Because Jesus told her *she* was.

The little girl in me, all she ever wanted was for her mom to get help and healing. She is the little girl who met you hiding in a closet with her baby. The one who was gonna hurt her own little girl with her unhealed wounds.

And I could have stayed in there, you know. I could have kept moving on, dealing with pain the way I was taught, running from feeling it. I could have kept it all a little secret with just me and my baby. But it wouldn't have been a secret for long because my pain would have spilled out sideways all over my kids' lives, my marriage, my friendships, and my dreams. It had already started to. I could so easily have passed my inherited wounds on to my kids.

My mom and I, we were the same. We both collided with wounds. We both hurt. We both hurt others with what hurt us. And we both needed healing.

And yet, I'm not my mom.

The only difference between my life and my mother's was that I ran toward my pain instead of away from it, trusting Jesus could heal me there. That changed my life and my daughter's.

And she was worth it again and again and again.

Bella's all grown up now. And she's beautiful, and she's kind, and she's strong, and well, I'm biased of course, but she is God's gift of redemption to me. Everything I would have wanted in a relationship with my mom, God gave to me in my daughter. And instead of needing a lot of healing like I did at her age, she is going out chasing others who need healing.

God helped me walk out of that closet, not just for me, but for my kids and their kids and their kids' kids. So I am pleading with you right now.

The people you love are pleading too.

When we first started out, I told you that every closet is an invitation. Every trigger, every broken heart, every lie uncovered, every altercation, every walk-in absent of peace is God's request for your presence. Every shriveled hand, every revealing receipt, every cold snub, every low score, every panic attack, every stone cast, every tear shed, every need to forgive, every "I'm not fine," every "If you had," every darned wounded collision is God inviting you to heal. His love can't bear to watch you shaking in the pain of old wounds, inflicting new ones.

You can keep running from your pain. You can numb it. You can pretend it's not there. But you and I both know all that does is hurt you and everyone you love. It's time to do the hardest, best thing you can ever do: It's time to *stretch*. No more acting like it's gonna go away. No more waiting for God's magic wand. No more thinking you're gonna wake up transformed on Tuesday. No more enabling the people around you, being an accomplice to unhealed wounds. And no more saying "Someday"—for the big things or the small.

When you stretch, it shows the people you love why they can stretch to heal too. When you run into pain, as hard and messy as it is, it promises them they're worth healing for. When you trust God can meet you there over and over again, it gives them a permission slip to do the same. Your yes to healing will halt the hurt you inherited. It will alter the trajectory of your children and their children. It will change all your collisions. It might even change the world. Because you being more whole will leave every hurt person you collide with more whole.

Your precious Jesus, the One who loves you with an indescribable, sacrificial, do-anything-for-you love, He is pleading with you most. He wants to mend and restore you, the people you care about most, and this world that is in desperate pain. He stands in the closet, He sits in the chair, He stops at the party, He waits on the hill, He shows up in the synagogue, He risks absolutely everything. His life, for yours. Do you hear His voice?

Jesus says *Today.*

Stretch.

This one move could change everything.

a blessing

If you got in my daughter's car, you'd most likely hear one song cranked up as loud as it could be. It's called "The Blessing." Some of the words you would belt out at the top of your lungs with Bella are

May His favor be upon you
And a thousand generations
And your family and your children
And their children and their children.[1]

And you'd sing this part over and over with bold faith, as though every line anchored the promise of God's goodness, saving, presence, and healing into the future reality of your people. If you asked my daughter why she thinks her story looks so radically different from my story and my mom's story and my grandmother's story, she would say, "Just listen to this song." I think what she is trying to say in anthem that she's not saying in words is *Because. Jesus.*

Years ago, when I sprinted into a closet to avoid my pain and the one who'd caused it, I could have sat in there and kept it all a little secret with just me and my baby. But it wouldn't have been a secret for long because my pain would have spilled out sideways. It had already started to. I could have so easily passed on to my kids the wounds I'd inherited. But Jesus crash-course collided right into my life and invited me to run into Him so I could heal. God helped me walk out of that closet for *my* kids and *their* kids and *their* kids.

Over the years, my kiddos have seen the good, the bad, and the ugly. I haven't hidden a thing. They know the trauma I went through, they know the mistakes I've made, they know my complicated relationship with my parents. They have seen me cry, beat myself up, go to therapy, get mad, and ugly grieve. Instead of pretending I was fine, I let them in on the truth that I needed Jesus' help and healing. And that might sound crazy to you, but it won't be the first time I've sounded crazy to you. (Duh, we met in a closet.)

Because my kids saw my real story and my real pain, they also saw my real Jesus show up and do a real healing. They witnessed Jesus start to use my pain, not my perfection, to help all these characters they have grown up around. They saw the way Jesus pursues broken people and loves them back together. I wouldn't trade their front-row tickets to learning compassion and empathy and authenticity and a need for God for anything. I don't believe for a second that because I have prayed or because I have sought the Lord, my kids won't have to trip and fall flat on their faces, stumbling to find Jesus just like I did. They don't inherit my faith. They choose their own. They do, however, have a head start and a strong foundation, and they know where they can run in their pain now too.

If you time traveled back to the generation before me and the one before that, the inheritance passed down to my children would look thick with addiction and thirst, wounded patterns and wreckage, neglect and imprisonment, absence, abandonment, godlessness, self-worship, pride, and dysfunction. My kids should be heirs of suffering, inheriting past pains like a legacy they are not proud to wear. And that's not to say that my kids don't have struggles or don't make mistakes or won't experience hardship, but the absolute truth that redemption is real and possible is seen in their lives every day.

I am utterly blown away by the grandiose possibility that Jesus Christ can intersect your pain and halt the generational wounds that have been passed to you. I am convinced that those wounds do not have to be handed down to your children or the people you love. I have seen the move of God, the power of God, the saving of God. It is possible, and it is yours for the taking.

The people you love most don't inherit your faith, but they do inherit what you did with your pain, who you ran to when you hurt, and the way your mess spilled out sideways and caused theirs. They also inherit the riches of what they experienced when you got well, paid attention to your grief, modeled that it's OK to get help, let people carry you, and got on your knees pleading for Jesus to come. This whole faith thing is not about not needing God; it's about needing Him. It's not about looking the part, checking a religious box, or saying all the right things. It's about colliding with Jesus over and over again because you desperately need Him for the good life. And when you experience the healing you long for, your loved ones inherit who to run to and how to get there when life hands *them* hurt.

So friend, the longing you have for your own life and the lives of those you love is possible. Jesus' healing, help, rescue, power, presence, and transformation are available all day, every day. Allow Him to collide with every aspect of your life. Let Him move in and take over. Let Him stitch you up and stitch you up again. Keep meeting Him at the well, on the chair, and along the way. The life you long for your children and their children to have has everything to do with how much *you* allow Jesus to intersect *your* life.

Jesus has legacy and love, healing and purpose for you and your people. In fact, God wants to bless you so you can be a blessing. Turn that song up if you need reminding. God wants to heal your pain and your people's pain so you can go out and help heal others. He wants to see you and your kids and their kids really make it count, bringing hope and healing to a broken world. He won't use your perfect family story, because you don't have one. He will use your "We need Jesus in our pain and brokenness and maybe you do too" story.

So friend, as my family rolls down the windows and sings at the top of our lungs to a world that needs what we do—Jesus' healing—we hope you can hear us:

He is with you . . .
He is for you . . .
Amen.[2]

The words of this blessing are already yours. *Because. Jesus.* Keep colliding, friend. This healing—it's for you and your children and their children.

xoxo,
Willow

amazed and amen

A Prayer of Surrender and Thanks

Jesus,

I am amazed by You. When I collide with Your life and allow You to run into mine, You astound me. You are more beautiful than I could have imagined, more wonderful than I could have understood. The more I spend time with You, the more I want to.

I recognize that I need You. I need Your rescue, and I need Your help. On my own, I have the great capacity to hurt my own life and the lives of others. I need You to be my Savior. Save me from selfish ambitions, self-sabotage, hidden strongholds, deep-seated lies, destructive patterns, wayward paths, twisted beliefs, and all the other things that get in the way of healthy relationships with You, others, and myself. I need rescue today and every day. Thank You for being my Rescuer and my Healer.

Please keep mending and restoring me. You know all the ways life has handed me hurt. I need You to stitch me back up and make me well again. I turn to You instead of all the other things I have turned to for healing. I know that You invite me to participate in the healing I long for. So here I am *today*, extending my life to You and inviting You into all the spaces and places within me that need You. I know

I have pushed You out, but I now give You permission to come into my pain and grief, my anger and my loneliness. I trust that You are safe and good and can take what is broken and make it so beautiful.

I am forever grateful that You took my shame, my wounds, and my mess upon Yourself. You showed me on the cross that there is nothing You wouldn't do for me. Your love blows me away. What can I do to pay You back? Thank You for Your promise that I don't have to. Your life for mine. May my life be a reflection of the gratitude I feel for what You have done for me.

Lord, I want to declare to You so that I may never forget: I belong to You, and I am so grateful that You belong to me. You are my Refuge, my Home, my Compass, my Rock. You are my Healer, my Help, my King, my Friend. To Your invitation to come and follow, I say yes.

I hand You everything I have and everything I don't. I surrender my past, my present, and my future. I hand You my body, my mind, my heart, and my soul. I entrust You with my strengths and my weaknesses. I even give You my disappointments and my dreams. I don't want to be anywhere else but where You are. Where You go, I will follow. Instill in me the courage it will take to walk into the places You enter and do the kind of work You do. Help me to be like You, Jesus, to my family, my friends, my neighbors, and everyone I collide with. Use me as I run toward people in pain to bring healing and help. Purpose me for Your glory and make my life really count.

In Your name, Jesus,

Amen.

discussion questions

Feel free to use these questions for your own growth and healing or for processing the ideas in discussions with a friend, a small group, or a book club.

Part 1: Running Away from Pain

1. In chapter 1, Willow says, "Every closet is an invitation. Every trigger, every broken heart, every lie uncovered, every altercation, every walk-in absent of peace is God's request for our presence. . . . It's often in these stuck places that we experience a real and personal, living and compassionate God, showing up and helping us get unstuck." In what ways are you sensing God's invitation even in the midst of your pain?
2. How have you been "schooled" to handle your hurt? (See chapter 2.) Were you told spiritual platitudes like "Pick yourself up by the bootstraps"? Were you shown how to be strong and pretend everything was fine? How has this gotten in the way of true healing?

3. Willow says we don't move on, we move *with*. That is, the pain we've experienced in our lives moves forward with us. (See chapter 3.) What pain or fear or coping mechanisms have you been moving *with*?
4. In chapter 4, Willow talks about ten of the many ways we try to heal ourselves. Which of these do you resonate with most? What has been the result?
5. In your own words, explain what Willow means by a "wounded collision." (See chapter 6.) In what ways can you see that your own unhealed wounds have been colliding with the wounds of others?

Part 2: Running Into a Healing God

1. Describe a time you told someone "I'm fine" when you were anything but fine. How could you have responded differently to let someone into your pain and allow them to help carry your burden?
2. What assumptions have you made about God based on your experiences with His people? How does the story of Jesus' collision with the woman about to be stoned help to change your assumptions? (See chapter 9.)
3. What pages of your life feel blank to you? Or what pages do you wish you could rewrite? What truth can you hold on to when you are grieving those blank pages?
4. As you've been reading through the stories in these chapters, what has Jesus been revealing to you about your own woundedness? What wells might you be drinking from that are

making you sick instead of satisfying your thirst? What areas of brokenness need healing?

5. In chapter 14, Willow says, "Often the belief you and I attach to brokenness in relationship is *I would be loved IF________.*" How would you fill in this blank? How have you filled in this blank in your relationship with God?

6. In chapter 16, Willow talks about survival instincts that might no longer be serving us but are keeping us stuck—we fight, we run away, or we freeze. Which of these responses do you find yourself falling into most often? How do you sense Jesus prompting you to move to get healing?

7. Review the *A-B-C* concept in chapter 17. What self-beliefs have been "bossing you around" and leading to more woundedness? What are some Post-it note truths you have picked up in this book that you can stick to yourself today?

8. Picture yourself among the people at the foot of the cross. (See chapter 19.) How does it strike you that all of your mess and wounds are on Jesus and so are the wounds and sins of those who hurt you most? Take the time, alone in prayer or in a journal or aloud in your group, to tell God how grateful you are for His love that promises "by his wounds we are healed."

Part 3: Running Toward Pain to Bring Healing

1. Willow says in chapter 21 that "healed people help heal people." She also acknowledges that running into people who are hurting can be scary. She reminds us that when we are not sure what to do, Jesus says, "Be Me." Name a few ways you could "be Jesus" in a difficult relationship in your life.

2. In chapter 22, Willow talks about purposing our pain—making it count for other people's healing. What are some ways you sense God might be able to use your own story of pain to bring healing to others?

3. Reflect on these words from chapter 23: "The work of loving others begins with allowing God's love to penetrate all the places and spaces within us that don't yet believe they are lovable." Are you loving others the way you want to? How do you feel about the idea that your lack of love for someone might be connected to your own belief that you are not lovable? What would change if you could see your lack of love as an indicator light reminding you to go to the Source of Love when you're having a hard time mustering up love for someone you collide with?

4. In Matthew 12, we see a man who longed for healing but who could have had all kinds of reasons to push it away. When have you found yourself feeling like accepting help and healing might cause more harm? How do you find yourself saying, "Someday"? When you see Jesus pressing in and suggesting healing *today*, what do you sense He wants to heal? How is He asking you to participate?

notes

Chapter 4: Not Dealing Is Not Healing

1. Mark 5:26.
2. William Barclay, *The Gospel of Mark*, The New Daily Study Bible (Westminster John Knox Press, 2001), 148.

Chapter 5: A Wounded Collision

1. "Property of Jesus," by Bob Dylan, track 3 on *Shot of Love*, Columbia Records, 1981, https://www.bobdylan.com/songs/property-jesus/.

Chapter 7: I'm Not Fines

1. See Mark 2:1-12.
2. Mark 2:3.
3. Galatians 6:2.
4. Mark 2:5.
5. Mark 2:5.
6. Mark 2:11.

Chapter 8: Drunkards, Gluttons, and Swingers

1. Matthew 11:19.
2. Luke 14:12-13, MSG.
3. See Mark 2:13-17.
4. James R. Edwards, *The Gospel According to Mark*, The Pillar New Testament Commentary (Eerdmans, 2002), 82–83.
5. William Barclay, *The Gospel of Matthew*, vol. 1, The New Daily Study Bible (Westminster John Knox Press, 2001), 333.

6. R. Kent Hughes, *John: That You May Believe* (Crossway Books, 1999), 405.
7. Mark 2:17.
8. Mark 2:17.

Chapter 9: Wanting to Be Wanted

1. Oscar Wilde, *Lady Windermere's Fan*, ed. Ian Small (Bloomsbury, 2014), 64.
2. See John 8:1-11.
3. William Robertson Nicoll, ed., *The Expositor's Greek Testament*, "Commentary on John 8," StudyLight.org, accessed April 29, 2025, https://www.studylight.org/commentaries/eng/egt/john-8.html.
4. Matthew 5:28.
5. Jeremiah 17:13.
6. John 8:10-11.
7. John 8:11, KJV.
8. Gerald L. Borchert, *John 1–11*, The New American Commentary, vol. 25A (B&H, 1996), 376.
9. William Barclay, *The Gospel of John*, vol. 2, The New Daily Study Bible Series (Westminster John Knox Press, 2001), 9.

Chapter 10: Absence Makes the Heart

1. *Collins Dictionary*, "prodigious," accessed March 17, 2025, https://www.collinsdictionary.com/us/dictionary/english/prodigious.
2. See Mark 5:21-34.
3. Mark 5:24.
4. Mark 5:30.
5. See Psalm 56:8; 139:13-16; Isaiah 43:1; Luke 12:7.
6. Mark 5:33.
7. Mark 5:34.
8. Psalm 147:4.
9. Chris Tomlin, vocalist, "Good Good Father," by Pat Barrett and Tony Brown, sixstepsrecords and Capitol CMG, 2014.

Chapter 11: Rescue

1. See Luke 15:1-7.
2. Luke 15:4.
3. See Luke 15:1-7.

Chapter 12: Thirst Traps

1. See John 4:1-42.
2. John 4:10.

Chapter 13: If You Hads

1. See John 11:1-33.
2. John 11:3.
3. John 11:4.
4. Barclay M. Newman and Eugene A. Nida, *A Handbook on the Gospel of John* (United Bible Societies, 1993), 375.
5. John 11:21.
6. John 11:25-26.
7. John 11:27, 32.
8. John 11:35.
9. See Isaiah 53:3.

Chapter 14: Reckless

1. See Luke 15:1-2, 11-32.
2. *Merriam-Webster Dictionary*, "prodigal," accessed March 9, 2023, https://www.merriam-webster.com/dictionary/prodigal.
3. See Leviticus 11:7-8.
4. Luke 15:17.
5. Luke 15:18-19.
6. Luke 15:20.

Chapter 15: The Over and Over Again

1. Matthew 18:21.
2. James Hastings, ed., "Forgiveness," *Dictionary of the New Testament*, StudyLight.org, accessed May 4, 2025, https://www.studylight.org/dictionaries/eng/hdn/f/forgiveness.html.
3. Matthew 18:22, NLT.
4. Barclay M. Newman and Philip C. Stine, *A Handbook on the Gospel of Matthew* (United Bible Societies, 1992), 577.
5. Warren W. Wiersbe, *The Bible Exposition Commentary: New Testament*, vol. 1 (Victor Books, 1989), 67.
6. See Matthew 18:23-35.
7. Craig S. Keener, *The IVP Bible Background Commentary: New Testament* (InterVarsity Press, 1993), 95.
8. Matthew 18:32-33.
9. Lewis B. Smedes, "Forgiveness: The Power to Change the Past," *Christianity Today*, January 7, 1983, 26. See C. S. Lewis Institute, accessed May 4, 2025, https://www.cslewisinstitute.org/wp-content/uploads/forgiveness.pdf.
10. Luke 23:34, ESV.

Chapter 16: Getting Unstuck

1. See John 5:1-18.
2. John 5:18, MSG.
3. James F. Strange, "Beth-Zatha (Place)," in *The Anchor Bible Dictionary*, vol. 1, ed. David Noel Freedman (Doubleday, 1992), 700–701.
4. Craig S. Keener, *The IVP Bible Background Commentary: New Testament* (InterVarsity Press, 1993), 275; John F. Walvoord and Roy B. Zuck, eds., *The Bible Knowledge Commentary: New Testament* (David C. Cook, 1983), 288–289.
5. Keener, *IVP Bible Background Commentary*, 275.
6. John 5:6.
7. Spiros Zodhiates, ed., *The Complete Word Study Dictionary: New Testament* (AMG, 2000).
8. John 5:7.
9. Mary West, "What Is the Fight, Flight, or Freeze Response?" Medical News Today, July 29, 2021, https://www.medicalnewstoday.com/articles/fight-flight-or-freeze-response.
10. John 5:8.
11. John 5:9.

Chapter 17: The Power of B

1. See Proverbs 23:7.
2. Psalm 139:14.
3. See Matthew 8:5-13.
4. Warren W. Wiersbe, *The Bible Exposition Commentary: New Testament*, vol. 1 (Victor Books, 1989), 33.
5. Bible Hub, "*kurios*," accessed May 12, 2025, https://biblehub.com/greek/2962.htm.
6. Matthew 8:8.
7. Matthew 8:8-9.
8. Matthew 8:10.

Chapter 18: Get Out of the Boat

1. See Mark 5:1-20.
2. "The Tombs," Bible Hub, accessed May 5, 2025, https://biblehub.com/topical/t/the_tombs.htm.
3. Mark 5:4-5.
4. Rick Knarr, "The Lord God Almighty," Sermons by Logos, 2022, https://sermons.logos.com/sermons/960775-the-lord-god-almighty.
5. Mark 5:7.

6. John F. Walvoord and Roy B. Zuck, eds., *The Bible Knowledge Commentary: New Testament* (David C. Cook, 1983), 123.
7. Mark 5:9.
8. Walvoord and Zuck, *Bible Knowledge Commentary*, 123.
9. Mark 5:15.
10. See Mark 4:35–Mark 5:2.
11. 1 Corinthians 11:24, MSG.

Chapter 19: The Ultimate Wounded Collision

1. "Matthew 8:17 Meaning," from H. D. M. Spence and Joseph S. Exell, eds., *The Pulpit Commentary*, King James Bible Online, accessed May 5, 2025, https://www.kingjamesbibleonline.org/Matthew-8-17_meaning/.
2. See John 19:28-29.
3. See Matthew 1:23.
4. Luke 23:46.
5. Luke 23:34, ESV.
6. Matthew 27:46, ESV.

Chapter 20: Get Off the Bus

1. If you'd like to know more about Ciderpress Lane, visit https://ciderpresslane.com.

Chapter 22: Make It Count

1. For more information, please visit Team Julia at https://www.teamjulia.org.
2. John 16:33.
3. See 1 Corinthians 11:23-25.
4. Allan Kellehear, "Dr. Elisabeth Kübler-Ross and the Five Stages of Grief," Elisabeth Kübler-Ross Foundation, accessed May 6, 2025, https://www.ekrfoundation.org/5-stages-of-grief/5-stages-grief/.
5. David Kessler, *Finding Meaning: The Sixth Stage of Grief* (Scribner, 2019): 9, 7, quoted in Jane E. Brody, "Making Meaning out of Grief," *New York Times*, November 4, 2019, https://www.nytimes.com/2019/11/04/well/mind/making-meaning-out-of-grief.html.

Chapter 23: Always

1. Matthew 22:37-39.
2. 1 John 4:19.
3. 1 John 4:7, 8.
4. *The Free Dictionary*, "vulnerable," accessed May 7, 2025, https://www.thefreedictionary.com/vulnerable.
5. C. S. Lewis, *The Four Loves* (Harcourt Brace, 1991), 121.

Chapter 24: The Yellow Butterflies

1. "Amazing Grace," by John Newton, 1779.
2. See Hebrews 11:1.

Chapter 25: Mended and Restored

1. See Matthew 12:1-14.
2. William Barclay, *The Gospel of Matthew*, vol. 2, The Daily Study Bible Series, rev. ed. (Westminster Press, 1975), 22–23.
3. Barclay, *The Gospel of Matthew*, vol. 2, 28.
4. Matthew 12:13.
5. Matthew 12:13.

A Blessing

1. Elevation Worship, Cody Carnes, and Kari Jobe, performers, "The Blessing," by Steven Furtick, Chris Brown, Cody Carnes, and Kari Jobe, track four on *Graves into Gardens (Live)*, Elevation Worship Records / Elevation Worship Publishing / Essential Music Publishing LLC, released May 1, 2020.
2. Elevation Worship, Carnes, and Jobe, "The Blessing."

acknowledgments

As I hold this book in my hands, the one I dreamed of, prayed over, wrestled with, hated, loved, and sweat for, I release it into the hands of God. I know full well any words I have to say that could possibly birth hope or faith or any life change at all are from Him. He is the One who chased me down, found me orphaned, brought me home, stitched me up, whispered my name, and called me His own. Without Christ crash-course colliding right straight into my broken life, my story would have no hope or help to impart. It's He who met me in my pain and He who uses me there. As I trust God for what He will do with this message, I am keenly aware that I could never have written it without Him.

I fully acknowledge that I am a thousand stories woven together by those I have collided with. I know full well that who I have become, and the work I have been given the opportunity to do, has everything to do with the people God has put on my path. This book is a reflection of their imprint and influence on my life.

To Rob, Aidan, and Bella, your presence in my life has brought healing, redemption, and family. Just you being you reminds me every day that God is indeed good and does keep His promises.

Deuteronomy declares, "GOD, your God, will restore everything you lost; he'll have compassion on you; he'll come back and pick up the pieces from all the places where you were scattered."* You three are proof that God truly restores what we've lost. I have been broken to pieces, but man, has God used you to put me back together. My heart and life are full because you're in them. Love you with all I've got.

To my friends who have become like family, you know who you are. We don't share a last name, but you feel like home. Thank you for being my people. I will weep, wonder, belly laugh, dance party, charcuterie, and stargaze with you any ol' time.

To the Collide community, with your bravery to be real about your pain and brokenness, your willingness to go with me to find healing in Jesus—you astound me. I have learned what it looks like to be authentic, to grieve, to name what is true. You have taught me the power of story, togetherness, and truth. You have shown me that we can hurt *and* we can hope. You have proven God can take what feels so very broken and make it astonishingly beautiful. Thank you for colliding with me.

To the women who sacrificed so this book could become a reality, thank you. Michelle Holladay, thank you for giving your days off for years to keep this dream alive. Without you I would have given up long ago. Thank you, Kristen Behrends. Doing this meaningful work with you will go down as one of my life's greatest gifts. To Breeze Potts, thank you for being the safest space to process life, faith, heartache, healing, mom life, vulnerability hangovers, and all the things.

To the team of amazing people who made this work possible: Anna Kuttel, Kim Taddonio, Ashley Sherron, Jaelyn Libolt, Brynn Paxton, Chloe Johnson, Kylie Cartagena, Kenna Warren, Kristen

* Deuteronomy 30:3, MSG.

Mattila-Dempsey, Theresa Butcher, Amanda Garvin, Carla Moore, Carol Ingram, Jamie and Lisa Imus, Aaron Nelson, Jon and Shannon Epps, Jermaine Larson, Laurie and Doug Bunnell. Thank you for what you did to get this message into the hands of women who need to be reminded that they are worthy of healing. For refining my writing and making me a better author—thank you, Deborah Beddoe and Leeana Tankersley. For believing in me—I am truly grateful to my agent Rebekah Von Lintel. For your mentorship, gems of wisdom, listening ears, and always pointing me toward Jesus, thank you, Donna Vandergriend, Pam Pries, and Gini Bunnell. For sitting in my pain and being Jesus' healing presence in this world, I am grateful for you, beautiful therapists Karolyn Merriman, Erik Johnson, and Margaret Manning-Shull. A huge shout-out to the Tyndale crew, Kara Leonino, and Donna Berg for working so hard to get these words into the world.

To my Cindy, who God used to save me, I miss you so, but I know you're making heaven a good ol' time. To my mom, your pain and love taught me so much. I am holding on to the great hope that I will one day see you happy and whole in heaven. Until then every butterfly gives me faith. And to my dad—we didn't get nearly enough pages. If it means anything, I wish I could have filled every last one with you in them. To my Uncle Rikky and my Aunt Rhonda, who gave me a home when I didn't have one, thank you will never be enough.

To my new friend who picked up this book: Thank you for allowing my story to collide with yours. I honor your heart to walk toward healing, and I am so grateful that the God who collided with my life is colliding with yours.

about the author

Willow Weston is an author, a speaker, a podcast host, and the founder of Collide, a ministry impacting women nationwide. With decades of experience, Willow brings passion and truth, sharing her own journey of pain to inspire others to invite Jesus into their brokenness so they, too, can experience healing. Willow leads conferences that empower, heal, and transform women. She has authored several Bible studies, including *The Birds and the Lilies*; *Personal and Powerful*; *Go Ahead*; *Yes, You*; and *Collide and Converse*.

Willow loves telling stories and inviting others to share theirs. She's a spelling bee champ but loses miserably in Trivial Pursuit. She can throw a mean dinner party but is a criminal at the local library. She has a hippie name and once lived on a school bus as a kid. Willow frequents coffee shops more than she'd like to admit and sits across from hurting people in the hope that they will find help for their pain. She uses china on Wednesdays and loves making the ordinary feel extraordinary. Willow battles insecurity and old wounds every day, just like you probably do too.

She collided with Jesus in college, and He became her direction, her healer, her hope, and her rescuer. Jesus met her in her brokenness and has used her there too. She's been married for more than twenty-five years and has two kids who teach her more about God and life than she could ever teach them. Willow is as real as you get, obsessed with hosting parties, coffee, the beach, and a good, good story.

JOIN WILLOW WESTON
TO ENCOUNTER JESUS IN A TRANSFORMATIVE WAY.

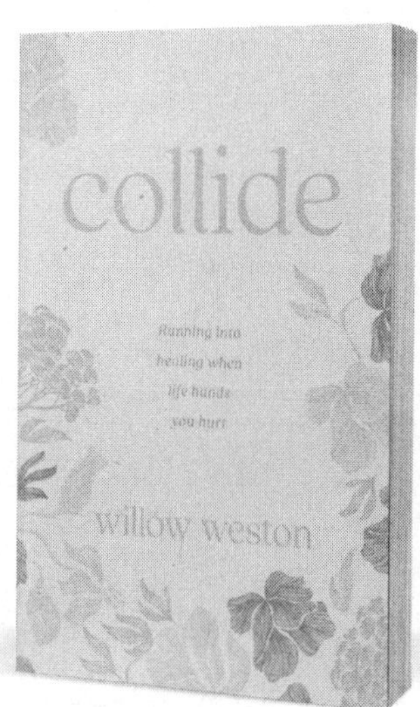

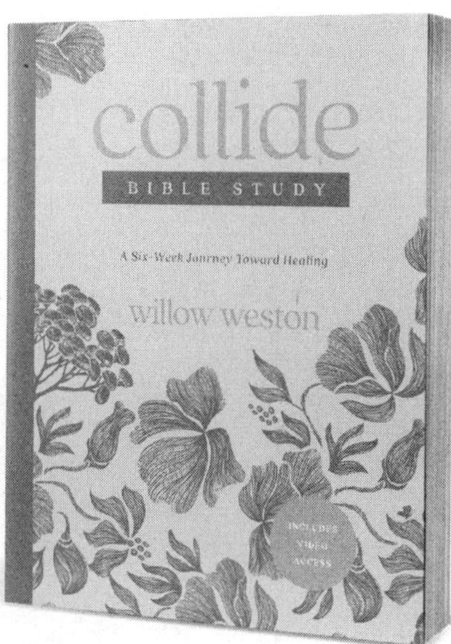

Collide is about knowing a God who doesn't run from pain but runs toward it, colliding into our wounds in a way that leaves us less broken and more whole. The more we collide with Him, the more healed we become; the more healed we become, the more healing we bring into all our collisions.

In the *Collide Bible Study*, Willow invites readers to encounter Jesus through the stories of biblical characters who experienced His help, healing, hope, and rescue, and we learn how to apply the same truths in our own lives.

AVAILABLE WHEREVER BOOKS ARE SOLD.

CP2080